Chasing Perfection:

A Journey to Healing, Fitness, and Self-Love

Rachel Brooks

Chasing Perfection:

A Journey to Healing, Fitness, and Self-Love

Rachel Brooks

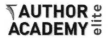

Identifiers:
LCCN: 2019913431
ISBN: 978-1-64085-914-2 (paperback)
ISBN: 978-1-64085-915-9 (hardback)
ISBN: 978-1-64085-916-6 (e-book)

Available in paperback, hardback, and e-book

Book design by JetLaunch.
Cover design by Debbie O'Byrne

Dedication

To my mother.

*"You have to be your own best friend first
before you can be someone else's."*

You were right.

The Story of the Butterfly

A man found a butterfly in its cocoon. He sat and watched the butterfly for hours as it struggled to force its body through the little hole at the end.

Eventually, the butterfly stopped making progress. It appeared as if it had gotten as far as possible, and it could go no farther. The man decided to help the butterfly, so he took a pair of scissors and snipped off the remaining bit of the cocoon. The butterfly now emerged easily, but it had a swollen body and small, shriveled wings.

The man continued to watch the butterfly. He expected that, at any moment, the wings would enlarge and expand, the body would contract, and the butterfly would flutter away. But that didn't happen. Instead, the butterfly spent the rest of its life crawling around with a swollen body and shriveled wings. It would never fly.

In his kindness and haste, what the man did not understand was that the struggle required for the butterfly to free itself of the cocoon's tiny opening were nature's way of forcing fluid from the body of the butterfly into its wings so that the butterfly would've been capable and ready for flight once it achieved its freedom. The struggle was necessary for it to achieve flight.

– **Author Unknown**

Table of Contents

Note to the Reader

Dear Reader,

Thank you for picking up a copy of *Chasing Perfection*. If you're like me, you're probably wondering, why this book? Maybe you, too, are a perfectionist, or you're looking for ways to cultivate self-love or recently embarked on a fitness journey of your own, or perhaps you'd like to know if the chase ends. Whatever the reason is, I hope you find it throughout my story.

So, why *Chasing Perfection*? I asked myself the same question. The best way I can answer that is, we're all chasing something. For me, I chased perfection. As silly as it sounds, now, without it, I wouldn't be where I'm at today, sharing the journey.

When writing a book was first suggested to me, I scoffed. Immediately, my guard went up, and I turned the suggestion down. I let fear decide and do the talking for me. *Who? Me? Write a book?*

The truth was, I was terrified. As I opened my mouth, my insecurities screamed, *I'm not a writer. I'm not an expert. I'm not good; I'm not this, that, and so on.* I believed the excuses to be valid, leading me to question and doubt myself. *Who am I?*

Who am I to share my story? Who am I to write a book? As much as I wrestled with this idea, the suggestion had planted a seed.

Who am I? Fear reminded me. Somewhere buried inside, I heard the same voice in a small whisper ask, *who are you not to share your story? If not you, then who?* Then, it hit me. If this is the same voice, why am I choosing to listen to the negative one? I believe we all struggle to decipher which voice to listen to, and the one I'd been choosing for most of my life was the one I fed—fear. It was then I decided differently. I chose positive over negative and saw the good in myself and my story.

As someone who chased perfection and other's highlight reels for way too long, I made a promise to myself to always show up, not just for myself but for others. I vowed to be as honest and transparent as possible, including what I share in this book. Spoiler alert—life isn't just the highs, and perfection doesn't exist.

We're all flawed. We're all perfectly imperfect, and as promised, I lay out what all of that looks like in the pages that follow.

While writing this book was one of the most challenging projects I've ever created, it was also a rewarding, therapeutic, and cathartic process—a labor of love.

Throughout *Chasing Perfection*, I share some of my deepest, darkest, most secretive, and heartbreaking moments, including ones that I've suppressed for years, as they were too painful to relive. These may trigger or be sensitive topics to some readers, so take note before diving in. There were times while writing that I got choked up while reading sections back, and parts that truly moved me. But this isn't just my story; it's a part of my story. To counter lows, we experience highs. I also share some of my best moments, the moments that bring me joy, make me grin from ear to ear, and still light me up—even to this day. This is all part of the journey of life—ebbs and flows, highs and lows, ups and downs.

Throughout this book, perhaps you'll find parts that resonate with you and your story. We are more alike than we are different, and I encourage you to take the lessons I've learned and use them to shortcut whatever you're going through. To know where we're headed, we must first understand where we've been. Through experiences of my own, I hope to give back and inspire, encourage, and empower you to embrace a life filled with passion and purpose.

As we go through life, we look for evidence to support our stories, lies, and beliefs, and for many, we don't take the time to address what's holding us back. Instead, we push it aside or add to our oversized, overweight baggage collection. Whatever we hold on to will continue to hold on to us. For years, I carted mine around, busting at the seams, unaware of what I'd carefully and cautiously packed away. While unpacking and sifting amongst my life's collections, I finally found what I'd been looking for. And even though everyone's journey is different, I hope your outcome is the same, to find what you've been chasing after.

I hope as you read this, you feel my underlying wish for you to become your best and most confident self. I wish you a life filled with incredible love, joy, peace, happiness, and freedom. I want you to achieve everything you want in life. My wishes for you are the same wishes I had for myself, but that's all they were—wishes.

I'm here today to tell you wishes do come true and not in some far off, fairytale way, but in a way in which your soul feels ignited from within. The dreams you've dreamt that felt way too big and scary, the life you silently watched as others live your dreams. All of those things are possible with action.

Although there are many takeaway lessons shared in this book, it's up to you to choose what to do with them. It's up to you to choose the outcome of your life. Everything comes down to the choices we make. What we choose will determine our destination. We have the power to choose truth over lies, love over hate, confidence over doubt, faith over fear, and courage over comfort.

These choices require courage to step up, be bold, be brave, and own who you are. If you desire more, you must change what you're currently doing. It means loving and accepting yourself. It means getting to the root of who you are and healing the wounds that hurt the most. It means letting go of what no longer serves you. It means no more shame, no more guilt, no more baggage. It means forgiving and setting yourself free.

You deserve more. I believe you were created to shine; you have to believe, though, or it will have no impact on your life. You must love yourself and know you're worth it. The key to unlocking your destiny is found in the power of your choices.

As I look back, I'm excited about the future. No matter where you are in life, whether it be your personal journey or fitness journey, I want more for you—you deserve more. You were destined for greatness!

Upon completion of *Chasing Perfection*, in 2018, I applied everything I've learned and teach throughout this book back onto the fitness competition stage and won! When you get out of your own way, you become unstoppable. This is the message

I hope you take from my story, and this book altogether—you have the power to create your own story.

Love yourself.
You are worth it.
You are enough.

XO,

Rachel

Introduction

I distinctly remember the first time I stepped into my silver hologram suit and heels to practice my posing for the 2012 bikini competition. I looked in the mirror and shuddered at the thought of what I'd gotten myself into. At that moment, I wanted to quit, but I'd made a commitment and was willing to do whatever it took, even if it meant putting myself on the line.

Now, four months later, I was standing backstage, looking into the crowd of 400-plus people cheering loudly. The lights were hot and bright, and the music and energy amped up. This was it; this was the moment I'd been waiting for. Practically naked, shaking in my five-inch heels and heart pounding, I listened for my number to be called. Suddenly, I felt embarrassed.

What was I thinking? Every insecurity was on display, every flaw exposed. How did I get here? Despite my small upper body, my thick legs dominated my frame, followed by my wide hips and butt to match. Although my stretch marks and cellulite were covered with layers of spray tan, they didn't feel hidden. I knew they were there, and that's all that mattered. Fundamentally, I hated myself, and now I was about to parade all my flaws on stage.

On public display, I felt naked and vulnerable. As much as I tried to walk in five-inch heels with grace and poise, my body language gave me away. I had zero confidence in myself, my body, or my presentation—everything was on the line.

Looking into the sea of hundreds of expectant people, I was at the mercy of the judges. I hoped all my hard work was enough. I hoped *I* was enough. That's all I could think. I was vulnerable—nowhere to hide, totally exposed. In a matter of minutes, my fate would be decided as I paraded my body across the stage to be judged.

Standing there, nervous, shaking, grinning a fake, cheesy smile, and waiting for the judges to give the command for the next pose, I knew deep down that I'd failed. I didn't belong here. I wasn't enough. It was at that moment, trying so hard to be something I was not, knowing my heart wasn't in it, that I felt myself fade. There was nothing I could do but finish and pretend everything was fine.

I had hoped that if I pretended to be someone else—if I wore the right masks, appeared as the person the judges wanted me to be—it would be worth the sacrifices. In my mind, it was all for the greater good.

After the prejudging, I knew I hadn't placed. I felt a heaviness inside. I left for our break and burst into tears as my inner critic raged ferociously. I could hear it above my sobs, *You knew you weren't good enough. What were you thinking? You were never going to win. You're not ready. Look at you, look at the other girls. They're so much better and prettier. If only you had pooped this morning, you'd have lost more weight; you'd be in the double digits. I can't believe you wasted people's time and money to come watch this. You're a loser and a failure.*

I didn't know it then, but I'd hit my all-time low. I was unaware that the consequences of my choices led me to that long, rocky road to hitting bottom—but all that would soon change.

ONE

The Makeup: One of the Boys

I grew up in the small, rural suburb outside of Buffalo, New York—population 3,500—with my eldest brother, Jason, middle brother, Jeremy, and youngest brother, John. My father was a self-employed woodworker and custom cabinetmaker, and my mother stayed home until the youngest was in school. She worked a series of jobs to help provide additional income for the family, eventually landing a service rep position at a major health insurance company.

Growing up, we didn't have much financially—very little for extras, and every cent was accounted for. On shopping trips, we'd be reminded of that whenever one of us—my brothers or I—added to the cart.

It wasn't until grade school that I noticed other kids had more. They wore new shoes and clothes throughout the year, took vacations, and even had the cool snacks packed in their lunches like Fruit Roll-Ups, Snack Pack pudding, and Little Debbie snack cakes. Sometimes, they'd be given money to buy treats after lunch like ice cream or pretzels. I wondered why we didn't have the means for such luxuries. Why were they able to afford extras when we couldn't?

When I was very young, I thought free lunches were cool, like I'd won something special. "Oh, you have to pay for your lunches," I'd say with a smile. "Not me, I get them for free." Once I realized what free lunches actually meant, I no longer felt special.

At an early age, I began comparing myself to others and wanted more. I hadn't considered myself to be different—until one day when I attended a birthday party.

I wanted to get my friend a Barbie doll for her birthday but was told we couldn't afford it. I looked over the knockoff, bargain version my mother told me to settle for. The doll was pretty, just like the other Barbies, *and* her hair grew. A smile emerged on my face. *She'll love it.*

My mother got the doll, and we wrapped it in the best paper we had. Then she drove me to the party. All the little girls were having a great time playing games, eating cake and ice cream, and the birthday girl opened her presents. I was eager for her to open mine. I wanted to show her the cool features. *Look, her hair grows!*

Sharing the moment with my classmates and friends, I watched with excitement as she opened present after present, all the toys I'd wished for on my Christmas and birthday lists. And then came a Barbie and the little girls were gleeful, oohing and aahing, including the birthday girl. A wave of disgust came over me, and I felt myself sink. The excitement quickly changed. My heart sped up, and my hands felt sweaty. In that instant, I wanted to disappear. I no longer wanted her to open my gift. I began to feel less than, embarrassed, and ashamed. *If only I could have gifted a Barbie.* Soon my gift was announced, "And this one is from Rachel!"

I hung my head as she opened the gift, and the glee from the little girls didn't explode as it did with the *real* Barbie. My friend still wore a smile from her previous gift as I tried to compensate and one-up the Barbie by telling her that the doll's hair grew. I wanted to belong and feel special too. "I love it, thank you," she said. I smiled but knew I couldn't compete. My gift was the *generic* Barbie. It wasn't good enough.

As the party came to an end, she thanked everyone for coming and for the gifts. She told me again how much she loved the doll as her mother sneered in front of me, "At least you have a *real Barbie* to play with." Seriously! What kind of person, let alone a mother, would belittle an already embarrassed child in front of her peers?

With that remark, my life was shaped, and a new perception of myself took hold. I was ashamed, embarrassed, and made to feel less-than in front of my classmates. My mother picked me up, and I couldn't wait to go home to cry. I couldn't comprehend what had happened exactly. All I knew was, whatever happened made me feel something I'd never felt before and never wanted to feel ever again. Pushing it away, I lied to my mother and told her what a good time I'd had and how my friend loved her gift (or maybe she just had better manners than her mother). I lied because my mother didn't need to feel my hurt too.

Experiencing this firsthand, I was determined to never, ever feel *less-than* again. I was ashamed of the pity others took on us, either directly or indirectly—my parents always did and gave the best they could. Still, it was the little digs in my early years that wounded me and shaped my character. I promised myself I'd work hard, so I'd never feel the pain of going without ever again.

Growing Up

It was the 1980s. Aside from my mother, I was the only girl in my family. I looked up to her for everything. When she wasn't at work, she was busy taking care of our household, carting us kids off to sports or events, always prioritizing the needs of her children and my father above herself. She was an excellent cook, and when I wasn't outside playing with my brothers and the neighborhood kids, I was by her side in the kitchen, watching her cook our family meals and bake treats for special occasions. Everything she made was a work of art and love. She's the most selfless person I've ever known.

My middle brother, Jeremy, and I were inseparable. Just two years older than me, we did everything together. He was my best friend. We'd play in the dirt with Matchbox cars and Micro Machines for hours, building cities and towns complete with tunnels and roadways. I loved being creative and using my imagination. We lived near a creek and would walk the banks talking for hours. We'd turn over rocks looking for crayfish, salamanders, or whatever slimy critters we could find to collect in our buckets.

I connected with boys more than girls because of my brothers. The act of being girly, dressing up, doing hair and makeup, gossiping, all the stuff that young girls do, was lost on me. In a houseful of masculinity, my mother and I were outnumbered; it was much easier to fit in than to stand apart. I was happy, and I belonged.

While growing up in the 80s and 90s, TV and magazines were my only sources for learning what women were *supposed* to do and look like, and it caused conflict within me. I didn't have much of a feminine influence or peers of my own. I occasionally toyed with wearing a girly outfit, applying makeup, and styling my hair, all of which I learned from admiring a male friend's older sister. She had the looks, the stylish big hair, trendy clothes, and knew the coolest music. It was fun and new, but at a young age, it didn't feel like me. So, I would go back to wearing one of my brother's shirts, wiping off the makeup, and pulling my hair in a ponytail. It was more comfortable hanging with the boys. It wasn't complicated.

The foundation for my self-image and self-esteem developed around the media. The women possessed a natural beauty and were portrayed as flawless and perfect. A soft glow radiated from their already perfect skin as they glided down the runway as models do. They were feminine, beautiful, tall, and elegant in their gorgeous chiffon dresses with ruffles and frills. I would have loved to wear a dress like that, but with my short, stocky body, I'd look like I was drowning inside a sleeping bag!

As grateful as I was to have had a loving family—always laughing, playing, and living a spirited childhood, there were shadows as well. When I was two years old, I was diagnosed with nephrotic syndrome, a kidney disorder, and spent most of my early years on prednisone. I had to avoid salty foods, check my protein levels, and pee a lot. When I started school, I looked and felt chunky and swollen from the water and sodium retention, as well as the steroid medication. I felt different compared to other kids and became self-conscious. At times, I couldn't partake in special treats because of the additional salt. I didn't like the unwanted attention, especially when my class had to wait on me while I peed. Eventually, I outgrew the kidney disorder, but I never forgot how it made me feel.

Unfortunately, my mother didn't have much of a feminine influence herself while growing up. She did the best she could to foster and teach me what little she had learned on her own. Raising a family—primarily of boys—she didn't value self-image as a priority.

As I grew older, these circumstances fueled my desire for perfection. Societal norms and rules confused me at an early age. I didn't like what I saw in the mirror—a short, plain-Jane tomboy. Why was it hard to play with or relate to other girls? Why did it feel forced and uncomfortable even though I had a longing for acceptance and belonging? I wanted attention and to be noticed for who I was, not because of my kidney disorder or because I hadn't brought the right kind of doll to the party. Anything about me that was unique felt wrong. I struggled internally to connect and belong. Overcoming this would become my life's journey.

On Femininity

It wasn't until adulthood that I learned or understood what it meant to be feminine. I did not achieve a sense of beauty, confidence, self-love, or self-worth that came from embracing one's softer side, one's light, and identity. When I was growing up, my mother and I didn't talk about feminine power or women's empowerment as we have now. As young women, we were on our own to find ourselves and our self-worth.

My family moved to the city, Buffalo, the start of my sophomore year of high school, and it marked the first time

I felt I belonged. I met amazing girls who asked me to hang with them. I wanted to dress and act like them. I felt like Tai from Clueless, the tomboy trying to fit in[1]. They were pretty and popular, and each had their own identity and place in the group, in school, and in sports. These were what I felt real girls looked and acted like. These were the girls I admired; I wanted to be them. It was a fresh start, a sneak peek into what I was missing, and I loved everything about it. It felt awkward at first, but I eagerly took to embracing this new role. Just as I was getting acclimated and embracing my new identity, we moved back to my small hometown the following year.

It was devastating to go back to being lost and confused. All the progress I'd made felt wasted. I'd just gotten comfortable with the new me, the feminine me. Now, I felt forced to revert to my old ways because I was too afraid of being rejected as my new self. I couldn't bear the thought of being shunned and rejected again. I was starving for attention, always wanting to be loved and accepted. I continued to play small, so I wouldn't stand out for the wrong reasons. I didn't want to be different again.

I always wondered what made these girls different—was it small-town life versus big-city life? Did their mothers and/or sisters grow up having examples of femininity and self-worth? How did they learn to own themselves? I was fascinated by the differences between those girls and me, but I also tormented myself with such thoughts.

When I compared my country life to city life, it was a stark contrast. I felt I belonged in the city, but I had no control over where our family lived. My encounter with femininity, self-care, self-worth, beauty, confidence, and identity had passed me by. I suddenly was at a loss for a community of like-minded females owning themselves, empowering others to be strong, beautiful, and confident. Till my year in the big city, I had no idea what I'd been missing, a place to fit in!

Exposed to that level of acceptance ignited something in me. Everywhere I looked, there were feminine influences. I wanted to be just like the models, my new friends, the other girls in school, anyone and everyone—except me. Although I was finding my way, I was still struggling. I hated what I saw in the mirror; it just wasn't enough. I'm not even sure what *enough* was, but I didn't feel whole and satisfied. Something was still missing.

A Moment for Gratitude

My parents were the most hardworking people I knew. Once my mother started working at a health insurance company, the additional income provided enough to allow for a few extras, including opportunities to play sports year-round. I loved soccer, even though I wasn't very good. It was great being part of a team. My parents gave to their children unconditionally and selflessly while working hard to provide. Although there were times when it was tough, we always had just what we needed. We never went without. We were happy and healthy. I can't thank my parents enough for everything they gave us, including the love, support, faith, and values they instilled. The struggles and hardships we experienced helped shape me into the person I am today, and for that, I am grateful and proud of my family.

For Safekeeping

I grew up knowing that no one is allowed to touch you in your private areas, and I was to tell my parents if this ever happened. But when it happened, I didn't tell them. It's not that I didn't know or understand it was wrong. It's because I was scared. The brains of small children aren't developed enough to make rational and logical decisions; they only recognize what is right and wrong. I did what I thought was best and kept my mouth shut for the sake of protecting my family and others. The fear of consequences led me, ultimately, to remain silent.

Keeping my secret safe, I buried it deep inside. I had no idea that it might fester, creating a mental and emotional prison. I grew into an ambitious young woman with my life ahead of me and no time to waste. And so, I plunged ahead into life and love, having no idea that the downside to my silence awaited me years down the road.

Points to Ponder

Be impeccable with your words. You have no idea the impact and scars your words will have or on whom they'll leave an impression, particularly when someone is in a fragile state. It might be a small child, who wants only to be accepted and appreciated.

I've learned that people will forget what you said,
people will forget what you did, but people will
never forget how you made them feel.
—Maya Angelou

TWO

The Crutch: Cloaked in Shame

Body dysmorphia is a term I learned later in life. I first heard about it while watching an episode of *What's Eating You?*. The young woman suffered from anorexia and had a hard time seeing her body for what it really is. She was sickly thin and ate nothing but a bowl of oatmeal. She had a warped perception of self-image, and so did I. Instantly, I was drawn to her and her story, and I felt a strong connection. I knew her struggle with self-image and eating disorders all too well.

During the show, a therapist asked the woman numerous questions, and I found myself relating to her answers. In particular, she caught my attention immediately when she asked, "What's your perception of your body?" She echoed my answer, "I think I look fat," she replied. The therapist then suggested a body tracing exercise to show the woman a different perspective of her body. She handed the woman a marker and a roll of white paper and instructed her to trace an outline of how she saw her body. The girl drew what she believed was true—a much larger outline of her body.

"Is this really how you see yourself?" the therapist questioned.

"Yes," the girl replied.

The therapist then instructed her to lie down on the drawing, and she began to trace the outline of the woman inside the borders of the drawing. The woman stood up and saw her reflection within the body she drew herself in. Tears filled her eyes as she now had a visual, and her perception of reality shifted. She realized that she'd convinced herself that she was much, much bigger than she really was. She suffered from body dysmorphia—and so did I.

* * *

I never saw a therapist because it would mean asking for help or admitting something (and maybe more) was wrong with me. Now, I'm all for seeking professional help, and I recommend it. But at the time, and by way of Google searches, I diagnosed myself. Body dysmorphic disorder became my new crutch— my new label.

What I found online became ingrained in my heart: People with body dysmorphic disorder have a distorted perspective of self. They fixate on their appearance, perceived flaws, and imperfections. They have difficulty controlling their negative thoughts, constantly compare how they look to others, seek approval and validation from others. Due to shame, anxiety, and embarrassment, they may avoid photos or social situations. Yep, I was that girl, almost happy with a diagnosis for my problem, though not a solution.

Comparison to other girls had gone back as far as grade school. I thought something was different and wrong with me.

started off too. My younger brother and I would look forward to sleepovers in the city, Buffalo, to spend time with our grandparents.

We stayed up late, enjoyed Nana's cooking—which was the best—and played well into the night with the neighborhood kids. I looked forward to summer mornings—waking up early on Saturdays, taking a break from the typical sibling rivalries over who got to eat the good cereal first, leaving the loser to eat Kix.

Nana made pancakes and sausage. For me, she made overcooked egg whites with the edges burnt just the way I liked them. It felt like a vacation. But that summer, one particular day, the vacation came to a crashing halt. All the excitement, innocence, joy, and laughter faded.

That Saturday morning, when I woke up, I felt dead inside. There wasn't anything to look forward to. I just wanted to go home to my mom.

Every night on these visits, my younger brother and I shared a bed. Exhausted from evenings of playing and laughing, we fell asleep with smiles on our faces, looking forward to another day of playing outside, exploring our imaginations and creativity.

On this night, laying on my left side, I heard someone come into the room. I assumed it was one of the adults checking on us. Drowsy and half-asleep from the long day, I was suddenly picked up and carried over someone's right shoulder, down the hallway to the left and into the back bedroom. With each step, I could feel my nightgown riding up.

In the guest room, I was placed in the middle of the bed on my right side, and as I lay there, in and out of sleep, easing into the comfort of this big, new, warm bed, I realized that someone had climbed in beside me. I kept my eyes closed, but my mind was fully awake.

My thoughts raced. *What is going on? This is wrong!*

As my mind reeled, I felt him slide up against me, spooning me, nuzzling into my neck and hair. I became instantly paralyzed. I was rigid, except for my eyes. *How could I get out of here?* I was crippled with fear! As he began caressing and breathing against me, his fingers started to make their way between my bare legs to my underwear.

Frozen, paralyzed, scared, confused, shocked, I lay there crying and praying that it would soon end. Seconds turned to minutes. Who knows how long it would have continued if there hadn't been an interruption from someone else in the house. God had saved me! I jumped up and ran from the bedroom, down the hallway, back into my bedroom, and buried myself under the blankets, shaking. I didn't want to wake anyone up. I didn't want anyone to know what had happened. I wasn't even sure what had happened. All I knew was that it was wrong … everything about it.

The next morning, I dreaded the long walk downstairs to face him, to see him, to see everyone else. I felt dirty and ashamed, like everyone knew; everyone knew that I'd done something terrible.

With no other choice, I made my way down to the kitchen and cautiously crept in, lingering at the doorway. Our eyes caught as my uncle (through marriage) gave me a look with his dark, beady eyes—a look of warning while my grandparents unsuspectingly tended to breakfast.

While looking into the open kitchen, a radical shift took place inside me. I felt my innocence and naivety lost forever. In an instant, I was forced to grow up while having a child's mind and body. At that moment, I knew I had a choice. Do I say something or not?

I recalled a conversation with my father one evening after a Bible teaching on heaven and hell—he told me he would do anything to protect his family.

"Even if that means going to jail?" I asked. "What about going to hell?"

To both, he answered, "Yes."

I knew my father loved me and would do whatever it took to protect me. In this situation, in my young mind, I knew my father would feel the need to protect me, and ultimately, he'd have to face the consequences. I wasn't ready to risk losing my father to jail or hell in exchange for this man and his actions. If I'd spoken out, it would have caused a ripple effect through my entire family. I knew someone would lose a father, and innocent lives would be ruined. I decided to keep my mouth shut. The secret burned within me for many, many years.

Looking back at that decision, I don't regret it. I do, however, regret not allowing myself to be the victim I needed to be. I masked this incident with excuses, hypotheticals, assumptions, scenarios—you name it. I tried to justify and rationalize what happened instead of facing what it really was—sexual abuse. The incident stole my youth and innocence and left me cloaked in a thick layer of shame and guilt. I wore it like armor. *Look at me—I'm so tough!*

Through my faith, I have forgiven my abuser, forgiven myself, and have gracefully and mercifully handed this over to God. No longer do I need to carry this heavy burden alone. It wasn't the act, in and of itself, that scarred me, but the mental and emotional damage that came with the act. The shame, guilt, secrecy, and lies kept me confined in an emotional prison.

* * *

Throughout high school, I was active in soccer. I thought playing sports and running would shape my body and trim my legs, but that didn't work. It only thickened my thighs with muscle, and I became more self-conscious to the point that I didn't enjoy playing. I wasn't very good at it anyway.

Another complex began.

I stopped wearing shorts.

And I began to think that if I ate less, maybe I'd get smaller, leaner legs and hips. So, I restricted food. At school, I'd limit my lunch to three Oreos. I also smoked cigarettes and drank endless cups of coffee to suppress my appetite. Dinner was whatever my mother made, and I ate it. Because by then … I was starving.

I kept trying to find extreme ways to manipulate my body with periods of food restrictions and binging—guilt, shame, punishment, repeat. If I wanted to lose a few pounds to fit into a pair of jeans, I just wouldn't eat. Simple as that.

Celebrity, glamour, and fitness magazines were unavoidable. They were everywhere and played on my vulnerable state of mind. I'd been beating myself up about not looking like the cover models since I was in high school. How did these women not have self-esteem issues? On the outside, they looked *together*, and their clothes fit their perfectly proportioned figures.

Meanwhile, my classmates appeared to be embracing their femininity with girly clothes. But I still held on to the Plain Jane, tomboy view of myself. I couldn't relate to girly girls. Needless to say, the combination of conflicting influences confused me.

My mind, body, and food issues left me feeling insec
and isolated. *Could I seriously be the only one? What is wrong
with me?* I carried my shameful self-loathing secret all alone.
I didn't want to live like this. I wanted to change but had no
idea how.

I chased this false ideal of perfection right onto the
competition stage. The only problem was that I was a prisoner
in my mind: trapped by my own distortions, living a life based
on self-inflicted fears, secrets, lies, and limiting beliefs. To prove
self-perceptions wrong, I pushed myself into the limelight. I'd
prove that Rachel was someone special and worthy of being
noticed—just watch.

I looked to the judges, complete strangers, for validation.
I needed them to say I was enough. The truth is and always
was that they didn't know me. They didn't know my struggles,
my pain, or my beliefs. They knew nothing about me. I took
all my shame, hidden body image issues, and baggage from
the past right onto the stage.

Today, I love my legs for many reasons. Simply put, I am
grateful I have them. It took me a long time and a lot of work
to get to this place of gratitude. When you sit and worry about
what you can or can't control in terms of your body features,
you are missing your bigger purpose in life.

When I worried about my legs, I missed out on wearing
shorts and dresses—the ways women did to embrace their
femininity. Now I recommend focusing on what you can
control, rather than finding lame excuses and throwing around
blame. Start documenting, taking pictures, or keeping a journal
on what you eat, what you wear, and how you feel in your most
vulnerable moments. Hold yourself accountable.

ng The Four Agreements by Don Miguel
oss a passage that really resonated with me[3]—
need to be accepted and to be loved by others,
cept and love ourselves. The more self-love we
have, the less we will experience self-abuse. Self-abuse comes from
self-rejection, and self-rejection comes from having an image of
what it means to be perfect and never measuring up to that ideal.
Our image of perfection is the reason we reject ourselves; it is why
we don't accept ourselves the way we are, and why we don't accept
others the way they are.

There will always be someone *more than you* ... more
beautiful, more confident, more successful, and so on.
Comparing yourself to others doesn't serve you; it will only
continue to hold you back from living a life of joy, happiness,
and love. While I wanted to know what it was like to be more
girly in school, I also wanted to be those girls rather than to
be myself.

Points to Ponder

What were the images of women around you as you grew up?

Growing up, did you identify more with the feminine or the masculine?

What parts of you today do you celebrate, and what parts do you feel confused about?

Was there an incident in your life that brought negative attention that caused you to hide?

* * *

Women can speak horribly about themselves. Have you ever heard your female friends speak in derogatory terms about their bodies? Have you heard yourself speak in this way about your own body?

- My lower body is huge!
- I hate my crooked smile.
- I'm not worthy of love.
- My butt is huge.
- I look like a centaur.
- People tell me I'm unique, but I feel *different*.
- I have a talent or gift that I think is weird.
- I can't go after my dreams because of _____.
- If I overeat, then I'll starve myself or excessively work it off.
- It's everyone else's fault I am like this.
- I can't talk about how I feel to anyone because it is embarrassing.

Cruel criticisms like these and many more have spewed from my mouth too. If any of these—or worse—criticisms sound like the narratives you play in your head, my question to you is:

**"What do you really want for yourself
if you could have it?"**

THREE

The Failure Cycle: Do More, Be More, Repeat

In my twenties, I thought I had my life together. Heading into this world as a *real adult*, I got busy and stayed busy. Out of high school and into college, I started working as a photo technician at a retail drugstore and quickly advanced into several management positions. I was good at it. After setting goals and accomplishing them, I received promotion after promotion. All I wanted to do was be the best at my job and make money.

At twenty-one, I was already a manager recognized within my district and asked by my district manager to relocate to open a new market in Columbus, Ohio. I was nervous but also excited about the freedom and adventure of being on my own. The opportunity was the exact challenge I needed. Moving was a considerable step outside my comfort zone—an effort to prove my worth again.

My job with the drugstore required a lot of physical and strenuous labor—bending, twisting, and heavy lifting.

At a young age, I experienced back issues. Straining my back, sadly, was part of the job, like a badge of honor. An orthopedic doctor diagnosed me with multilevel degenerative disc disease of the lumbar spine. He summarized that if I didn't start taking better care of my health, I'd be in a wheelchair by forty.

Leaving the doctor's office that day, I was shocked and overwhelmed by the heavy diagnosis he'd just dropped on me, but most of all, I was scared. Immediately I called my mother and broke the news. Her heart broke with mine, and I could hear the worries and fears in her voice as she tried to comfort me. She listened to my cries and reminded me of how strong I am. I wasn't sure if it was anger, fear, or my mother's belief in me, but it was the spark I needed; that was the moment I decided to change my life. The only problem was that I had no idea where or how to begin. Mentally and emotionally exhausted, I felt like my brain was about to explode. I started with what I thought was best; I threw away all the boxes of Hamburger Helper in my kitchen and dug out the offer for a free gym membership from the junk drawer.

In addition to work and health concerns, I was also attending school full-time to earn my bachelor's degree in business studies while working forty-five hours per week. I went to four different schools in five years. I started by majoring in business marketing with a minor in psychology, but after my sophomore year, I transferred to Buffalo State College, where that major wasn't offered.

If the above sounds like a lot, well, it was. I was making sure there was no time to think, and while my work and social life were thriving, school was hard for me to enjoy. It didn't excite me. The rewards were not so obvious.

Although school was a major priority, I didn't give it my best effort. I attributed this to one of my many self-limiting beliefs—I am not smart enough. As with all self-fulfilling prophecies, I did not perform well. I was also a social introvert. Without the crutch of a friend or knowing someone else in the class, connections with other students were hard to make. Working in groups was a challenge as I didn't feel I belonged or had anything to offer. *Why would anyone like me or want to work with me?*

After my move to Ohio, I was failing my third and fourth school, so my employer and I agreed to a transfer. I moved back home to Buffalo and graduated. I waited around a year for a then-boyfriend to finish his degree.

Before I knew it, I turned twenty-three. My boyfriend and I made plans to go back to Columbus together so I could finish what I'd started years earlier—work hard, get promoted, and be recognized for my success within the company. My head was full of visions of a new life with my boyfriend and a rewarding job—the whole perfect package. The only problem was, my boyfriend had no intention of moving to Columbus or being with me. He ended our two-year relationship, leaving me alone in Columbus with a broken heart and empty promises.

He was no different than any other boyfriend I'd had throughout high school and college. They didn't value me, and I felt worthless after every breakup. As a people pleaser, I gave my power to others and let them determine their happiness through me.

I didn't understand the concept of self-worth and boundaries based on my own values. The projected ugliness I felt outward, naturally, attracted men looking to take advantage of me. I felt completely powerless and had no idea what that meant at the time. They treated me poorly, with no love or respect. How could I blame them? I did the same thing to myself; I just wasn't seeing it. I got what I deserved, even though I didn't deserve it.

If I had known then what I know now, I wouldn't have settled for that crap. My experiences with men during this time compounded the pain and confirmed the self-limiting beliefs of who and what I'd become. Cumulatively, these relationships proved to me that no one would ever love me or want me, that I would never be good enough.

I tried so hard to prove my worth to these undeserving boyfriends; it was a desperate cry for love and acceptance. I'd see these attractive guys with beautiful girls and wonder what do these women have that I don't have? I'd compare myself. They were gorgeous, and had tall, lean bodies—overall, I believed they were better than me. Everywhere I looked—work, school, the media—I was inundated by their beauty and reminded of how much I didn't resemble this ideal. I never considered this as an extreme viewpoint. It was all I saw.

The fitness magazines caught my attention with promised headlines such as "how to get the body of your dreams" or whatever marketing jargon gained the most sales. Desperate to find the answers to my lifelong questions, I readily flipped through the pages. I thought that if I did the same squat and core workouts and ate the same diet, then I, too, would look just like the cover model. It seemed pretty simple. *I could do that!* But I continued to fail at even the simplest tasks and returned to what I knew best: extremes.

After my perceived failure, I'd eat a meal that left me bloated and feeling fluffy. The people on TV had killer abs, so I assumed that if they got them using the *As Seen on TV* ab roller, then I would too. I bought it. Each day I busted out a hundred crunches hoping to lessen the feelings of disgust and leave me with a rock-hard, flat stomach, just like the commercial promised. I was the perfect gullible customer—a sucker who fell victim to the newest and latest fads.

While working at the drugstore, self-improvement products were at my disposal. But I found myself to be an even more miserable failure. *Why was this so hard?* They were giving away the secrets, the "how-to" tips, and I still couldn't get this right!

I didn't have any real structure, and the notion of self-improvement greatly contrasted with my current lifestyle. Any sudden change was bound to set me back. Still, I was determined to find a way. The issue seemed to be that I didn't have the knowledge or tools yet to get there. I wanted help and change and was determined to find it.

Only this time, I was alone, without the boyfriend. I poured my heart and emotions into my work in an attempt to prove my worth. I put in my time, sixteen-hour-plus days, only to go back to my apartment feeling sad and lonely. My only forms of comfort were my cat (William), boxed wine, and cigarettes. I'd watch true crime shows and cried myself to sleep only to wake up and repeat the cycle all over again. I just wanted what I'd come here for—to get promoted and then leave.

Every day was the same—sad and depressing.

By this time, I was making more money than I'd ever had, and it was exciting. It was something of my own; I felt accomplished. I thought my promotions and my financial status would make me happy. I thought they would define me as successful. Success was a quality I admired in others—something I measured by status and wealth. Yet what I saw in myself was still a sad, lost person who didn't know where she was headed. I had no one to share my financial success with and, ultimately, felt betrayed by my boyfriend and friends. The thought of going through life alone was taxing and miserable.

Most of my life, I lived in the shadows of my brothers and others. They received attention for their skills, gifts, talents, looks, and connections. I played second fiddle and let them have the limelight and attention. The less focus on me, I thought, the better. But as the years carried on, not only did I get lost in those shadows, I got lost within. I lost myself.

I felt I stood out in a negative way. I relied on people noticing me—or not noticing me—to define myself. Outside of other people's behavior toward me and their validation of my worth, I had no other sense of myself.

Where was my inherent happiness?

I'd visit my family and friends back home in Buffalo any chance I'd get. Unlike in Columbus, I felt a connection and a sense of belonging in Buffalo. On one of my many trips back home, I flew to New York City to visit my oldest brother, Jason. The city made my soul feel alive. The intensity, bright lights, sounds, the hustle and bustle, the fast pace—I felt at home. It was during this trip that I made a decision. After my promotion in Columbus, I'd transfer and relocate to a drugstore near Jason. And as a do-over, I'd go back to school and get my MBA. The mundane life in Ohio was sucking my soul. This new plan allowed me to feel alive, have family nearby, and start my life over on my terms—whatever that even meant.

Upon my return to Columbus, feeling fresh and giddy, I had something to look forward to. Just ten more months, and I was out of there! Still, that was almost a year to fill, and I needed to feel better about myself. I joined the local gym hoping to meet people outside of work, make friends, build my own community, and find a sense of belonging. But I'd look in the mirror and think, *I don't even look good enough to go to the gym*. Everything about me was screaming insecurity and low self-confidence, and it showed in how I carried myself.

I sucked it up and went to the gym. As a newbie, I did what most women do—bypass the weights and head to the cardio machines. I thought if I started running, I'd get a lean, toned body, and I'd be skinny.

According to the magazines, "Skinny Is the New Sexy," and I wanted to be skinny *and* sexy. Then, maybe I'd find someone who'd love me. I stepped on the treadmill and hustled hard! My short, thick legs were pounding and thudding desperately to keep up. I was grunting and snorting, just trying to catch my breath. My heart was beating so fast; I could feel it through my chest. I thought I was about to die! My goal was to complete one mile. It was a start.

My heart was pounding, my lungs were on fire, and my face was tomato red, but I'd done it! I completed one mile in ten minutes. Even though I'd done it, I hated it! It felt awful. *How the hell do people do this? This is crazy!* No one was running like me. I was creating a scene with all the thudding and sound effects, and I felt so embarrassed! I couldn't even run right!

Afterward, I'd go home and wallow in my self-induced misery, and whip up a box of something or other, and cut myself down. *I'm such a loser and a failure.*

While this is painful to reflect upon, it is key in my message to young people trying to discover themselves in the gym. There is no cookie-cutter ideal workout for everyone's body. You need to exercise in a way that complements who you are.

Determined to find an answer to this fitness riddle, I continued searching; every failed attempt left me feeling worse. Why did this exercise stuff have to be so hard? I mean, I couldn't even master the next step after walking … running. *Wow! Isn't there anything I can do right?*

The irony is I love to work out now; it is my daily joy. But in my twenties, the attempts to be like other people were killing me and setting me up for failure down the road.

It never even occurred to me to touch the equipment at the gym aside from the ab cruncher—six-packs were in. All the cover models sported these beautiful, ripped abs, and were super lean. Remember, that's how the ab roller infomercial had sold me. With my limited insight, I stuck to the gym corner filled with cardio and ab machines and ate once a day. I assumed I needed to monitor my caloric intake and use the simple formula of calories in, calories out, to reach my fitness goal.

It seemed attainable enough, but it wasn't working. Did I need to run more or do more sit-ups? I wasn't sure, but there was no way I'd set foot in the weight area; I'd just be in the way and be a burden.

I already felt like an inconvenience in the lives of other people, so why would the gym be any different? Besides, the pretty cover girls' perfect bodies couldn't possibly have come from lifting weights. I believed lifting weights made you bulky and look like a man. And the last thing I needed was to get any bigger and bulkier.

That's why all the men were over there, not the women. Intimidated by the men lifting weights and thwarted by a lack of confidence—in myself and experience in the gym—left me feeling small and less than.

If only I had someone who knew what they were doing (i.e. *someone at the gym I could look up to and who seemed to have had their life together, looked good on the outside, a model or mentor). Somebody that I could aspire to be.*

I wanted to know how they did it, but even if a mentor showed up, I'd be too embarrassed to approach them. I just knew I didn't want what I had or to be who I was. If only the information and resources were as easily accessible as they are today.

The current generation is bombarded with the same distorted messages of perfection that messed with my head, but with the internet, they have a greater opportunity to learn and connect to others. They can watch videos, webinars, and read books. I heard people speak about overcoming self-defeating mindsets through attending events, workshops, conferences, and seminars. They learned how to make significant changes, internally and externally. They have a better chance of making an impact on the world by embodying positive behaviors like self-acceptance, self-care, and self-love.

I consider mine a cautionary tale for people who don't take advantage of all the information and support that is available.

Boyfriends No More

When you least expect it, life throws you a curveball. Shortly after my return to Columbus from New York City, I was feeling excited about my new plan to relocate after my promotion. I would go back to school and live in a city that lit me up.

One day, this guy walked into my work and headed to the freezer section. Stopped dead in my tracks, I found myself staring at him—something I'd never, *ever* done before. I'm way too shy for that. Besides, I'd never pursued anyone; I convinced myself such assertiveness would end in a letdown. But this time was different. I wasn't even aware I was staring until he saw my reflection in the freezer door and turned around.

Busted! There's no way I could fake the "I wasn't staring at you" look, so I played it off the best I knew how. I approached him, face blushed, stuttered some words, and tried to be as professional as possible. After all, I was the manager in charge of the store. I extended my hand and introduced myself. As he shook it, he informed me that he was our new ice cream vendor and sales rep. Hoping he couldn't see my nervousness, I tried to keep it together and act as businesslike as possible. After he left, I hid in the office until my nerves settled, and the redness subsided from my face.

OMG, I thought, *that was excruciating and embarrassing. I must have looked like a total fool. I've never felt or done anything like that before!*

* * *

"He's about to call you," a coworker said.

Instantly, the butterflies fluttered in my stomach. *I can't believe it!* "He's going to call me?" *Eek!* I sat at the counter in the pharmacy, waiting for his call.

My cell phone rang.

"I'm on break," I shouted back to the pharmacist as I ran out of the store. "Stay calm," I told myself.

Short of breath from my quick sprint, I answered the call as I unlocked my car door.

"Hello?"

It was him, the cute ice cream guy from the freezer section who I'd first seen in my store four weeks ago. He was calling me! Every nerve-ending in my body jumped with excitement and joy. Sitting in my Honda Civic, I nervously grabbed a cigarette to calm down as he took the lead in the conversation.

"Tonight?" I asked. "No, I don't have any plans." I lied. My evening plans of chilling at home with a bottomless glass of wine, and watching *Investigative Discoveries* reruns, with my handsome cat, could wait. *I can't blow this. He's THE one!*

After sorting the details of our date, I hung up. Staring at the phone in my hand as if it were a foreign object and this was a dream, still grinning from ear to ear, it suddenly hit me! *I just got asked out to dinner … tonight!* Immediate panic set in. *What will I wear? I haven't been on a real date in forever, and I'm so nervous!* I called my coworker to give her the details, and we shared in my excitement. I left work shortly after the call. I had better things on my mind.

On my drive home, I took a mental inventory of what I had that fit and looked decent enough for a date without screaming business casual or clubbing. Apparently, I only lived in those two extremes—hard work and hard play.

After a tall glass of Franzia White Zinfandel, I hopped in the shower and took my time; I needed to look perfect! Eventually, I settled on an outfit somewhere in the middle, a cute sweater and jeans with black boots. Giving myself one last glance, *Eh, it'll have to do, I can't be late,* I headed out the door.

The butterflies in my stomach were flapping away as I drove the short distance to the restaurant. I smoked another cigarette to calm the nerves, spritzed myself with perfume, and unwrapped a piece of Wrigley's Spearmint gum for a few quick, breath-freshening chomps.

I wanted to make a good first impression by being on time. Glancing around the restaurant, I saw he'd already been seated next to the door. "Am I late?" I said to myself as I checked my wristwatch. No, he'd just arrived early.

Making eye contact, he smiled and waved. I made my way through the standing crowd and greeted him with a nervous smile as I slid into the booth across from him.

We chatted about our call from earlier and laughed at how both of our coworkers were trying to set us up. He was easy to talk to, and I felt comfortable in his presence.

The waitress took our orders. I played it safe and ordered a simple cheeseburger, fries, and a glass of water, knowing I wouldn't eat much of it. I hated eating in front of people, specifically ones I was trying to impress. He ordered a steak, potato, and a beer. In between conversations, I picked at my food while he ate his meal. After dinner, he paid the bill and walked me to my car.

As I was leaving, I began to feel down and afraid that I'd blown it, and it showed. I tried to play it off as being tired, but I was actually disappointed. *That's it? This whole date is*

FOUR

Poker Face: Love and Loss

On a hot July day, my younger brother John, his girlfriend at the time, and I attended the annual Taste of Buffalo, the largest two-day food festival in the United States. Culinary experts from Buffalo and the surrounding area had gathered to showcase their top dishes and serve up more than two hundred specialties.

We were looking forward to trying new foods and enjoying the beautiful summer day with no reservations. The streets were lined with thousands of locals: food lovers, vendors, and attendees from across the nation. We made our way through the crowd and purchased a stack of tickets. The smoke from the meats cooking on the grills tantalized our taste buds. We were like kids in a candy store—ready to eat!

"Where should we start?" I asked, trying to look up and down the street. All I could see were the backs of the people crammed in front of me.

We stepped off the street and onto the sidewalk, opened a map, and began strategizing our afternoon. "We go to this place first," John pointed. "Then, we'll make our way down here." He said and pointed again. We all agreed and inched our way through the crowd. I didn't care where we started. I was just excited to eat!

Being short has its perks. Although I couldn't see above the crowd, I could easily squeeze my way through it, leading the way for the group. Standing in line, we each agreed to order something different and share, making the most of our time and tickets. We had an efficient system. Moving through the crowd from station to station allowed us to hit many places in the shortest amount of time.

The summers in Buffalo are perfect, a nice offset from the brutally long winters. I wore my white T-shirt and cobalt-blue shorts, and because the place was so packed, I opted out of carrying a purse.

I shoved my tickets, money, and phone into my right front pocket and made sure it was secured throughout the festival. The streets were bumping with laughter, chatter, street musicians, and filled with smiling, happy faces. You couldn't help but feel the joy and positive energy. As I satisfied my appetite at each station, I began to relax and give in to the lightness of this beautiful and perfect day.

We made our way to the Indian food stand and ordered tandoori chicken skewers, rice pudding, and a curry dish. Then, we stepped to the side to enjoy our bites. I felt vibrations on my right side. *Was that the music or my phone?*

Reaching into my pocket, I could feel my phone buzzing. I pulled out my Blackberry and saw "Dad" come across the screen. I answered immediately. "Dad, I can't hear anything. We're at the festival. Let me call you right back." I hung up— no point in trying to shout a conversation back and forth in all this noise.

"Who was that?" John asked.

"Dad," I replied. "Did he try calling you too?"

John pulled his phone from his pocket and saw that he had missed a call as well. We both gave each other a knowing look. We'd call him back in a minute. We had only a few bites left and had to move away from the crowd.

A few seconds later, while still holding my phone, it buzzed. It was Dad again; his words were something I will always remember, "He's dead." Everything in me sank. I dropped my dish, looked at John, and handed him the phone.

"What. The ..." I started. At that moment, time froze, and everything had gone pitch dark. The noises ceased, and in my mind, I was left standing on a desolate street with just my brother at my side. Everyone and everything had disappeared. Alone. Just the two of us. A few seconds later, reality set back in as the three of us pushed through the crowd, trying to get to a quieter area. The whole time, I kept telling myself, *No, no, no! This can't be. He can't be. What's going on? No, no, NOOOO!*

As soon as we were far enough from the crowd, I pulled out my phone and called my dad back. "Dad, what happened?" As tears filled my eyes, I held my breath as he replied, "We don't know." He and my mother were on their way. I braced myself against the cold, hard, brick wall. I slid to the ground and sat with my head in my hands. My whole world shattered at that very instant. This was real. My brother Jeremy was dead.

Meanwhile, people were happily making their way through the buildings, getting into their cars, filling the parking lot with laughter that bounced off the brick walls and looking back at us with curiosity.

"Keep walking!" I shouted at their happy, smiling faces. "Yeah, go enjoy your perfect life!" I choked the words out between sobs.

As tears of black mascara streamed down my face, staining my white shirt, I looked up to see John being comforted by his girlfriend. I felt so alone at the moment. I just wanted my brother Jeremy. He was always there for me.

Just a few days prior, I'd told him I loved him. If only I could say those words to him again. I wished I could let him know why and just how much he meant to me. His death was a sudden and shocking loss. After numerous investigations, we still do not have closure.

My protector and best friend, Jeremy, was a shining star and athlete, and he gave me unconditional love and attention. As a kid, I found my identity in him and followed in his shadow. I wanted to be like him—gifted, talented and loved by many. He showed me affection and attention, and he understood me. I never felt that I needed to be anything or anyone else when I was with him. He shined his light on me, and I felt noticed, like I was somebody special.

When he passed in 2010, at the age of thirty-one, the world as I'd known it had gone from twilight to complete darkness. I believed no one would ever love me or understand me as he did. When he died, so did a part of me.

After the Loss

Unfortunately, nothing I could ever do would bring Jeremy back. I was forced to learn a new way to live and grieve my own way. I did that in the best way I knew how, which involved distractions and not talking about it. I sought ways to push through, to change my life, and above all, to not feel. That radical decision eventually led me to the competitive stage.

Talking about emotions didn't come easy for me, including the passing of my brother. Other than a deep longing for his presence, I couldn't articulate exactly how I felt. There was an overall sense of emptiness, sadness, and loss. Life as I knew it would never be the same. His loss, the event itself, became the fulcrum of my life: there was my life pre-Jeremy's death and now, my life post-Jeremy's death.

Many nights I spent alone in a dark room, crying in pain, longing for my brother. I wanted to stay connected to him by trying to process the whys and hows, and learning to begin again. I had some major life-changing decisions to make. I needed to take a long, hard look at who I was and how I'd gotten to this point.

No longer did I want this to be my story. I didn't want sympathy. I didn't want to be the girl whose brother died— *poor thing*. "I'm stronger because of this." I thought. I had to overcome a loss that shook the foundation of my world. I held my emotions in and let them harden inside while I wore a new "everything's fine" mask. It fit perfectly.

Losing my brother would be the chink in my armor. I didn't realize how much of a lifeline he had been to me until I tried to fly solo without him. While I had Chuck in my life at this point and professional success, I was now raw and vulnerable from Jeremy's death. Any situation that could expose my broken parts, like an imperfect body in comparison to what was portrayed as acceptable, led me into a state of anxiety.

In the summer of 2011, one year after Jeremy passed, my girlfriends and I made plans to enjoy a hot day at the fitness center's pool. Sure, I was happy for the chance to get together and catch up from the busyness of everyday life, but I dreaded summer. My obsession with perfection and the sheer thought of anything *fitness*, *swimsuit*, or *body* related, left me feeling insecure and exposed. As part of the cycle to protect myself, I armored up so I wouldn't reveal my hurting insides on my outside. I did what I did best—I faked it. I spent years trying to perfect and manipulate my body and weight. I had the perfect system and plan—double up on my workouts, skip dinner, and take some poop pills the evening before. I'd wake up to an empty stomach, skip breakfast, and pray my belly would be flat enough to sit poolside in my two-piece suit.

I spent the rest of the morning mulling over which of my two swimsuits would make me look and feel my best. Neither satisfied, so I settled on the black one. Black is slimming; *let's see if it can slim my body into this season's sought-after beach and bikini-body*. Unfortunately, my summer body was my everyday body, and my everyday body was the one I hated. According to the magazines, it looked nothing like what it was supposed to. This summer would be a letdown—a reminder, again, of failing to reach my goals. As the pressure of yet another delusional expectation fell short, my self-judgment turned up the volume, deafening me with sour self-talk that dominated me my whole life.

My friends never knew I lived this way. I never told them. I understand now that holding back deprived us of having a very intimate and honest conversation—one I wouldn't hesitate to have with a group of women today. What if one of my friends was equally suffering? It was more critical to me to keep my body shame a silent secret and do whatever it took to make it through the outing.

On route, my girlfriends and I stopped at the store to grab a bite to eat. At this point, my stomach was aching with hunger. I thought, *Well, we're at the store that sells whole foods, I should be able to eat anything I want. After all, isn't that what you're supposed to eat?* I had no nutritional education regarding *what* to eat, *how* to eat, or *how much* to eat. All I knew was media, magazines, the Internet, and diets all said, "Eat whole foods." I walked in, hoping to find a snack to fit the requirements of what I should eat, but with so many choices, I became confused. I didn't know where, what, or how to begin. The bombardment of labels, such as whole foods, zero, diet, healthy, natural, organic, vegan, low carb, low fat, gluten-free, fat-free, sugar-free, cage-free, dairy-free, and so on, left me feeling overwhelmed.

After a few minutes mindlessly walking up and down the aisles, I settled on a small bag of chocolate chip cookies. Instantly, I became triggered by the word *cookies*. Cookies = BAD. *Nope. Can't get them. I don't want to have to run these off tomorrow.* As I was about to place the package back on the shelf, I noticed the bag's labeling: "whole grains, low fat, gluten-free, and vegan." I thought, *These can't be bad if they're omitting all the bad ingredients, and surely, I'm at a store that sells whole foods. These cookies could be good for me.*

Pleased with my label rationalization, I made my purchase. I felt confident in my decision until I noticed the other girls' snacks included *healthy* food options like veggies and hummus. Suddenly, I felt out of place, and my confidence turned to self-doubt. Immediately I regretted my decision, but the voices in my head told me otherwise, reminding me that I hadn't eaten since yesterday, and I did two workouts the day before ... I *deserved* these cookies. Agreeing with myself, I bit into the cookie and was once again pleased with my decision. They were so soft and chewy; I couldn't believe they were good for you!

I finished my cookie and added the rest of the package to my already overstuffed beach bag filled with the summer essentials and must-haves—tanning oil, sunglasses, water bottle, and the latest editions of celebrity, fitness, and beauty magazines—and we made our way to the pool. I couldn't wait to catch up with my friends and hear how their summers were going.

We sat poolside, and as I sat slumped over, I watched as my midsection folded like an accordion. Looking down, all I saw were rolls, and instantly, my mind was taken away from whatever my friends were chatting about and fixated on my body. Mentally, I checked out and left the conversation; I was too embarrassed and needed to fix this before others saw it too. I sat straight up, then back and watched as each position changed the number of rolls and thickness of each one. I was used to position playing and found the most uncomfortable ways to look my best and least rolly—it was painful. I'd arch my back, keeping my midsection stretched and taut, abs slightly flexed, holding my breath, my chest and chin up, arms and wrists positioned behind me. It was just enough to give the illusion of a sexy collarbone and shoulder pop. As I leaned back, the pain from contorting and all my weight pressed into my twisted palms. I turned my gaze downward as a half-smile smirked across my face. There, I did it! No rolls ... poised just so and afraid to move, or I'd ruin the illusion I created. The brief excitement of this ridiculous achievement quickly turned to disgust. It hurt. I hurt. Everything hurt.

Why is this so hard?

I exhaled a huge sigh of relief as I assumed my natural position, slumped forward, and tucked the bottom roll into my bikini bottoms. *There!* It's the best I can do, and I exhaled another sigh ... of defeat this time.

Looking for a quick distraction, I reached into my bag and pulled out a magazine—the *how-to's* for getting the perfect summer body, the perfect tan, wearing the perfect bikini, hosting the perfect party, and so on—basically, how to curate the perfect life. With the turn of each page, my anxiety heightened, and I began to feel less than. My distraction quickly turned to overwhelm. In a frenzy, I found myself comparing to see how I measured up with these beautiful, perfect images. I felt myself on the brink of emotionally shutting down. Determined I would not be a damper to any party with my hypercritical mind, I closed the magazine, picked my head up, and looked around. I saw inspiration and motivation everywhere. Fit, happy, healthy people surrounded me. I wanted to be like them.

The sounds of excitement and laughter pulled me out of my self-induced pity party. Everyone was laughing and enjoying themselves. There were squeals of joy as the young kids played and splashed around in the pool. And here I was, too focused on myself, wondering what others might think, and if they, too, saw my rolls, and were laughing at me? My insecurity had reached a new level, and the only way I knew to combat this feeling was to compare myself to someone in *worse condition*. I needed a boost of confidence, a high. It instantly made me feel better about myself, but as quickly as it came, it went. I was desperate for my next quick fix; I'd become obsessed. I was addicted, and I didn't even know it.

Desperate to lessen the feeling of defeat and self-loathing, I found myself judging, comparing, and criticizing myself and others. I knew better. I *was* better. Yet, I was sitting poolside at the fitness center, feet dangling in the water, the sun beating off my sweaty, oily body, thinking, the darker my tan gets, it'll help burn fat, and I'll appear smaller. After all, isn't that what tanning is *supposed* to do?

I scanned the crowd, and my eyes caught a young woman. The first thing I noticed was her midsection, also exposed, hers was larger than mine. Immediately, I felt better about myself. *At least I don't look like her,* I thought.

She was also with a group of girls, but she was doing something I wasn't. She was smiling, chatting away, and carrying on with what appeared to be genuine happiness and not letting her body get in the way of what really mattered— life. And I wanted to be her.

This should be me, enjoying my company, but I couldn't get past my flaws and insecurities. I couldn't let go of who I was. Much of my time was spent obsessing over how I looked and comparing myself to others. I missed the moments that mattered and often asked those around me how I measured up. I needed validation that *they,* too, saw my flaws and imperfections. Day by day, my body dysmorphia continued to grow as I fueled it with lies and comparisons.

Feeling defeated, I reached into my bag and grabbed a cookie. "Might as well," I muttered as I took a bite and watched the crumbs fall onto my sweaty, oily, accordion-shaped stomach. I hung my head and chewed slowly, as tears stung my eyes. *What am I doing? What's wrong with me?*

I had hit a new low. Taking in my surroundings, I saw fit people everywhere. I made assumptions about their lives based on their bodies. I intentionally sought the most unfit, so I could make myself feel better by internally putting others down. No one knew it, another secret I'd keep for myself. At that moment, I thought about my brother. He died, and this is what he left behind? A broken sister who spends her time criticizing herself and others? Through his passing, I suddenly had a glimmer of desire to do more and be more.

Overwhelmed with sadness, loss, and grief, this roller coaster of emotions continued as I attempted to pick up the broken pieces and "figure life out." I wanted peace. In an attempt at finding the silver lining, I chose to see my brother's loss as a huge wake-up call, proving life is too short and fragile. I no longer wanted to take mine for granted, living negatively. I wanted to make him proud. Not only did I need to be mentally and emotionally strong on the inside, but I also wanted to be physically strong on the outside, without a mask. It was hard pretending.

I didn't have a plan. So, I turned to what physically moved me—fitness. I used the pain of the loss as a driver and motivator to push through, hoping to cope and heal. I took action and did something more for myself. I joined the same gym my friends and I attended a few weeks prior. The motivation and drive were there ... the *how-to's* would be learned.

I thought if I focused on what I could control, I would get closer to my goal of filling this new hole in my life—a void of love, peace, and happiness. Aware of how fragile life was, I was determined. I started my health journey, and I didn't stop.

Pushing myself harder, faster, and further, the need to perform and be perfect left me struggling. I failed at the simplest tasks, such as running. I looked down at myself for this because my friends were avid runners, and they were skinny! Today, I can accept that I hate running and don't need to do it. But back then, I was in denial. This time, I told myself it would be different. I had a new goal: to create a new me.

Unfortunately, I still didn't have the insight or awareness to know why I wanted to create a new me. I only knew I wanted to be happy and look like the beautiful celebrities and fitness I longed to be like in my younger days. I hoped that this external goal and the satisfaction of reaching it would somehow help fill the void of Jeremy's absence. I acted tough on the outside so everyone would think I was strong, but on the inside, I just wanted to be happy, loved, and find peace with myself. I understand now, grieving Jeremy's loss was what finally set me on a long, arduous journey to becoming Rachel.

Knowing it would take time and hard work, I was prepared. With my new membership, I hired a personal trainer at the gym. He held me accountable and encouraged me to push through the discomfort when it got tough, and I wanted to give up. It was hard work! On a bright note, after six months of consistently working with my trainer, I fell in love with it all—the gym, community, and weightlifting.

Soon after that, I signed up for a fitness competition. While competing wasn't a happy chapter in my life, the decision to enter the competition paved the way toward making me who I am in the gym today.

We don't get to plan when life throws us lessons or the speed in which we learn them. This particular juncture in my life was supposed to include the fitness competition. It had to happen, and I had to fail hard to reap the wisdom gained from it.

Checking the application entry box, I immediately felt accomplished! *This is going to be awesome!* I didn't realize it at the time, but I was looking for a quick fix, a solution to a lifetime of self-hatred and dislike for my body.

Points to Ponder

Who do you allow to make you feel inferior or that what you have to offer isn't of value?

What exercises do you currently do in the gym that you genuinely don't like?

In what ways are you putting yourself through misery in your workout just to *check the box*?

If you are unsure, why are you doing it? Is it just because someone else does it?

What form of physical activity lights you up and brings you joy?

FIVE

Best I Ever Had: Where's the Peanut Butter?

By 2010, Chuck and I were married and had launched an internet start-up. I'd left my position as store manager at the retail drugstore long ago. After nine years and four promotions, my career at the drugstore chain had boosted me to a top position. Chuck and I were now living and working together pretty much day in and day out. Although we had our challenges, life together had romance and teamwork at its core.

Leading up to the 2012 Ohio Natural Bodybuilding Competition, I trained, dieted, and posed through an entire sixteen weeks of contest prep. Devoted to the competition and proving I could do this, I committed and sacrificed my life to do what it took.

Waking up early each morning, I kept to a strict regimen. My days consisted of eating every few hours and performing some variation of physical exercise, such as strength training, cardio, kickboxing, walking, and hiking. The idea was to keep moving. Some days included double workouts and extreme training sessions. If I wasn't dripping wet with sweat, I wasn't pushing hard enough. If I wasn't sore the next day, I hadn't worked hard enough.

Nothing was ever enough. Push, perfect, repeat—strive for perfection was my routine. This period led me to believe that the harder I pushed myself, the better I would be. *I'll have the body of my dreams and be so happy. Everyone will love me. Then, it will be enough; I will be enough.* And the chase would end. Finally, I could rest.

It was not supposed to be easy. If it were, everyone would be doing it. The more I sacrificed, the more I perfected, and the more value I invested, the bigger the reward. I kept telling myself this competition was for me and to prove my self-worth, not only to me but to others. I wanted to prove that I was *someone.* I convinced myself that eventually, in this process, I would stop hating myself. I would finally have everything I ever wanted: the perfect body, love, happiness, and acceptance—the perfect life. Well, that was the plan.

As the weeks passed by, I was visibly getting smaller, leaner, and withering away; even my boobs started to look like deflated water balloons. Halfway through prep, my menstrual cycle stopped, which was a new milestone—lean, but not lean enough. While my measurements, clothes, and scale reflected change, I couldn't *see* the changes. My body was changing, but my mindset was the same. Underneath, I was still a hopeless, sad person. "Stick to the process," I reminded myself, "and it will be worth it."

In the final week of training, I gave it my all, *a last chance workout.* As I was finishing up the last superset of trap-bar deadlifts with cable-glute kickbacks, I heard a pop come from my upper-right glute area. Completing the set, I headed into the final posing class. The whole time something felt off, and I kept kneading and massaging my upper glute. *I'll just deal with it later,* I thought. *Nothing* was standing in the way of this competition.

A week earlier, while practicing my posing, another competitor had pointed at my legs.

"Look at your legs," she said, looking me up and down.

Immediately, I shut down and became defensive. That voice in my head was laughing. *I told you they were huge, and now she's mocking you.* "What about them?" I snapped.

"I'd kill for those sweeps," she said with a smile.

I softened, let down my guard an inch, and thanked her. I wanted to accept her compliment, but this was a competition. *Was she trying to make me nervous? Was she toying with my mind? Or was she overly cocky?* I was already an emotional mess full of insecurities, and my inner critic would not shut up! I wasn't prepared to hear compliments, let alone process them. I was already too insecure. *You are nothing,* the voice reminded me.

Waking up on the morning of the show and having lost the final pounds of water weight, I made my way to get the final layer of my spray tan and have my makeup done. *Maybe this will be the moment I've been waiting for. Surely, now, I will look beautiful.* I looked at my gaunt face and saw only a stranger staring back at me. Colored with spray-tan and over the top makeup, I had become someone else. I felt the tension and anxiety rise as I rushed through the stressful morning. I looked forward to getting my hair done—going all-out with the long, dark extensions and creating the perfect curls.

The package was complete. Standing in my heels, dressed in my gorgeous bikini with blinged jewelry, I took another look at the one hundred-point-six pounds on my petite five-foot-one-inch frame. *Nope! It still wasn't enough.* I started to cry.

I didn't even recognize myself. *Who was this person? Who am I?* I was a mess, but again, I prepared myself, put on my mask, and pretended that everything was fine. I needed to be strong, brave, bold, courageous, and beautiful, even though I felt none of them. I had to suck it up. It was time for the show.

I felt the tears well up and did everything to hold them back. I couldn't let them ruin my makeup and streak my tanned face. As the host called the bikini division to the stage, we lined up numerically and walked single file across the stage. There wasn't any order. Short and tall, we had it all.

As soon as we took our places on stage, I could hear the supportive crowd shout their favorites, hoping to gain the judges' attention. "Let's go, number ten," "You've got this, twenty-three!" "Smile, fifteen!"

I held my forced smile, trying to get the judges' attention with my bling and posing. *Pick me!* Meanwhile, my heart was pounding while I tried to slow my breathing. *I'm so nervous, look at the judges.* Then my eyes met the crowd. *Shit!* My heart skipped, and the nerves shifted into overdrive. Shaking in my clear platform heels, I tried everything I could at the moment to calm down, breathe, smile, make eye contact, look sexy, be sexy, breathe, repeat. I felt so desperate, as if I were selling myself—cheap and fake.

I recognized a few people from my gym sitting in the front row and thought they were there to support me until I heard them shout the other girls' numbers. My heart sank, and my smile faded. I lost hope. Watching the judges take notice of other girls, I knew I didn't stand a chance. Nervous turned into downright pissed! *Just get me offstage. Where's the fucking peanut butter?*

I sobbed throughout my meal break—everything I wanted and had worked so hard for turned out to be a huge disappointment. During the finals, pissed off, full of rage and anger, I was determined to prove my worth once again. *I'll show them. Watch me!* While standing backstage for a second time, waiting to be called, this time my heart raced with adrenaline, not nerves.

I walked on stage to Drake's "Best I Ever Had" with such an attitude and sass, nailing my poses, glaring at the judges[4]. I shot them looks of sheer disgust. *Fuck you! How dare you not pick me!* Once I exited the stage, the adrenaline subsided, and I wondered, *Who was that girl on stage, and where did she come from?* One could easily mistake that attitude for one of confidence and self-worth. On the contrary, it was a defense mechanism. In a last-ditch effort fueled by adrenaline, determination, and shame, I still had something to prove—my worth.

Just as the results predicted earlier in the day, the stage filled with five beautiful girls, none of whom were me. According to my perfect plan, I was supposed to be up there with them. However, my physique wasn't what the judges were looking for, and that bruised my ego. I was hurt, exhausted, and once the nerves and adrenaline settled, I felt the physical burning and the throbbing pain in my glute. I just wanted to go home and hide. I felt like a loser and a failure. Now, I was officially embarrassed.

My family and friends left after finals. I apologized for inconveniencing them and for not placing. Now that the day was over, I was looking forward to eating pizza and drinking wine for the first time in sixteen weeks. *At least that should bring me comfort and make up for this horrible day.*

The pizza was burnt, and the wine was awful.

So, I turned to the nearly five pounds of Reese's I'd collected from each missed holiday over the last sixteen weeks and binged. The chocolate and peanut butter satisfied my soul. I ate until my insides felt like they mirrored my outside—a gross loser—and headed to bed.

The next day, I replayed the horrible event, and I was no longer safe from myself. I beat myself up. The hatred and negative self-talk were louder and stronger. I tried soothing my sad, crying soul again with Reese's, but it wasn't enough. Laying on the couch, feeling sorry for myself, I listened to Eminem's "Beautiful[5]" ironically, the words were hauntingly beautiful and fitting. At that moment, thinking this would be a great idea, I decided to go for a run to burn off the Reese's—hoping I would feel better. Even though it was just a competition, I just couldn't shake it. This was a big mistake. I was trying to erase the guilt of bingeing by running—the same pattern I'd repeated my whole life. I thought I could banish my childhood body issues by winning a competition.

It was an unseasonably hot morning that day. I was still dehydrated, exhausted, and in so much physical pain. I was about a mile in when I started burping up Reese's and on the verge of puking and passing out from the heat and exhaustion. Disgust and disappointment consumed me in every way.

Points to Ponder

In what ways are you living life to the fullest?

In what ways are you too trusting of others to know what is best for you?

What are you fighting to prove?

Do you find yourself easily offended? Why do you think that is?

What belief triggers you to react?

SIX

The Beautiful Disaster: Pitfalls of Paradise

The disappointment of losing the competition took a back seat to the constant throbbing, burning, and tingling in my upper glute area. I knew something was very wrong. Muscle pulls and lower back issues were nothing new to me. Actually, they were quite common, but this sensation was new altogether. I continued nursing the soreness, as I'd done in the past, by taking ibuprofen, hot baths, and applying a heating pad. I assumed the pain would go away on its own. It would have to. Chuck and I had our anniversary vacation coming up in a couple of weeks, and I didn't have time to deal with this. I was in such denial. As I continued to ignore my body's alarms, the pain worsened.

Eventually, the tingling made its way down to the sole of my right foot, which became numb. I walked awkwardly, and my right foot didn't snap back, it dragged. Blind and ignorant, I kept pushing through the pain. I didn't know what to do or how to care for myself. Since I couldn't see the gravity of the situation, a friend voiced her concern and suggested I make an appointment with an orthopedic as soon as possible.

To satisfy others' concerns and ease my own curiosity, I made an appointment. The orthopedic doctor pulled my chart and reviewed an MRI that was at least two years old. Based on a history of degenerative disc disease and my pre-existing low back condition, he determined my L4-L5 spinal discs were herniated. He advised me to get a cortisone injection immediately to relieve the pain. I scheduled an appointment for the same week.

I left the office puzzled. How could the doctor so quickly determine a diagnosis for my injury without a current MRI? After all, it was outdated. Was he even sure it was my back? I scheduled the injection for a few days later, but the decision didn't sit right with me. My gut instinct knew something was wrong.

That little voice inside, that gut instinct that loved me enough to call out something that could harm me, eventually saved me.

With the upcoming trip and the doctor's hasty treatment plan, I canceled the appointment. I didn't want to ruin or jeopardize my anniversary trip with Chuck, so I spent the rest of the week packing and nursing my injury. At this point, the excitement of this much-needed vacation to Las Vegas and Maui was my only focus. How bad could the pain be while having fun and laying in the sun? I wanted to make sure my husband was happy and try to forget the disaster of the competition.

The flight to Las Vegas was over four hours, and I could not sit still. My leg was burning, pinching, and tingling. I couldn't wait to land to walk it off. Walking seemed to be the only real reprieve at this point; it helped loosen my muscles that were tight from the flight and kept me moving. I needed to be strong—no time for drama. I was moving on from the competition. *Let's have fun. You'll get over it*, I kept telling myself, and I tried to make the most of our first evening in Las Vegas. The next morning, I gave myself a good stretch before sliding my legs over the bed. As I stood, my right leg gave out, and I fell into the wall. I couldn't feel the floor. My foot was completely numb!

Hoping I didn't wake Chuck, I gathered myself and sat quietly on the side of the bed, processing this new pain as a ball of emotions swelled in my chest. I was afraid of disappointing Chuck, more so than myself. I sat silently as tears welled in my eyes. *Why was this happening?! Why me?! Hadn't I had enough hurt, pain, and setbacks?* The sun was starting to peek through the shades, and I looked around the room with tear-filled eyes.

In my mind, this moment was the epicenter of a beautiful disaster. Amidst my internal conflicts of emotions, confusion, and chaos, I felt a hush of peace. All was still and quiet except for the pounding of my heart and the deep, heavy breaths of my husband as he slept. If only I could have stayed there, forever frozen, and not face all that would soon take place.

I fought back the urge to sob and stumbled into the bathroom where I sat on the cold marble floor and bawled. This wasn't part of the plan. We were at our favorite hotel and had planned to see a Cirque du Soleil show that evening with dinner at a fancy steakhouse. Everything was supposed to be perfect. I still had not recovered from the devastating loss of my brother, and now, with the loss of this competition, my pain and self-hatred pushed me to deny self-care. If only

I had done something differently, but I hadn't, and the result was this physical and crippling pain that cut into my soul.

After the release of emotions, I pulled myself together and wondered what to do next. How was I supposed to go about this trip without letting Chuck down? I had to be strong. My willingness to strive and my stubbornness not to admit pain left me wearing another mask. *Suck it up like you always do. That's who you are, a people pleaser,* said the voice in my head that ruled over me. It was true; people-pleasing was one of my defining characteristics—one day, I would have to change this to better myself.

I mustered through the few days of dinner and shows while in Las Vegas for the sake of my husband; there was no point in having both of us miss the fun. Maui was what I was looking forward to most for our anniversary. I was worried and scared I'd make the same mistake again in Maui, so I maxed out my allotted pain pills just to get as comfortable as possible for what seemed to be the longest flight ever! When we arrived, the pain I felt was unbearable, but I diverted my attention to the majestic scenery. It was breathtaking—both the view and my pain. It was the worst vacation in paradise you could imagine. My entire right side from the hip down burned, and my foot went numb. The pain was excruciating as I fought hard to hold back the tears. *Let's see how I feel in the morning,* I told myself. *We're in Maui—let's not ruin it.*

Waking up to another devastating morning left me crushed. I had no choice; I had to stop pretending and fess up to Chuck. So, I did. And as he listened, his expression shifted from elation to dead seriousness.

"This is so much worse than I've been telling you," I admitted.

While he was clearly disappointed, he took charge of the situation, which allowed me (for one of the first times in my life) to be taken care of. It was a glimmer of what a partnership could be like if you let yourself surrender (though it would take us another five years to get to that place fully).

Dragging my right foot everywhere I went, we found a doctor's office at a nearby hotel. Before I could get any relief, I had to endure the pain of simply walking. Admitting the seriousness of my injury, asking for help, and exposing my vulnerability made the situation worse. Letting my guard down crushed my ego; suddenly, I wasn't so tough! I half-listened to their diagnosis and given a shot for the pain. That's all I cared about. *Numb it, make it go away.*

As I stood up, I turned white and almost passed out from the pain and medicine. No longer in denial, I wanted the vacation to end, so I could be home and take proper care of my injury. There was no more ignoring this reality. Chuck and I were in limbo here, despite it being Maui.

On our last day, the doctor gave me enough medicine to make the burning and aching subside. I wasn't dragging my foot anymore. He wanted me to be as comfortable as possible for the long flight home to Ohio. And while it was the best I'd felt in weeks, I was exhausted in every way.

I had an appointment with my primary doctor the next day. She took one look at me and ordered an MRI for my lower back. As it turned out, I had ruptured my L5-S1 disc, and the rupture was pressing on my sciatic nerve. A million thoughts and questions ran through my mind as guilt and shame consumed me. My inner critic yelled at me for neglecting my body, ignoring the alarms, and carrying on with the competition even after I'd heard the *pop*.

I was truly disappointed with myself, but hey, I was in my favorite place—self-abuse. I caused this; I did this to myself. It was all my fault! Everything I tried to do, I failed. *I am a failure. I am a loser. I am stupid. I am careless.* The cycle of self-abuse dominated with every thought, punishing me over … and over … and over. Back down the hole of self-loathing, misery, and self-induced depression, I went. *Woe is me. I am the victim!*

Now I had confirmation. The plan was to treat it as fast as possible while avoiding surgery. I was scared. After all, I was dealing with a ruptured disc pressing on a major nerve. I tried to go back to the orthopedic with the current MRI, and they refused to see me because I had denied the doctor's order of the L4-L5 injection. I'm glad I didn't follow through. Who knows what might have happened had they injected this area blindly without a current MRI and into the wrong disc when the injury was L5-S1.

Over the course of four months post-competition, I experienced every form of treatment available, including steroids, pain pills, muscle relaxers, massage therapy, physical therapy, a chiropractor, and cortisone injections. Nothing worked, and only a few provided temporary relief. In a few painful months, my short-lived identity of a bikini competitor had gone up in smoke. The body I'd worked so long and hard at achieving no longer existed. All the weight I lost, I gained it back, plus more—twenty-seven percent, to be exact. The steroids made me hungry, swell, and retain water, and I felt bigger and grosser than ever. My metabolism was all messed up. Afraid to eat and gain more weight, I allowed the pain pills to help suppress my appetite. I thought they'd knock me out too—but nope, nothing. So, I added alcohol. That didn't do it either.

When dealing with a major nerve such as the sciatic, there is no masking the pain. It's still there, throbbing, burning, numbing, and tingling. The pills only provided a short relief, long enough to take a nap and be awakened by the same feelings. This was my new life.

The constant state of fatigue left me with a crushed physical and emotional core. I would pray and read but couldn't concentrate long enough to distract myself from the pain. I would go from my bed to my couch, to my office floor, just seeking comfort. The days and nights blurred together. During those four months, the discomfort of being in my body and the severity of the pain consumed me. My husband would have friends over, trying to have a normal life, and I would make a brief appearance wearing days-old pajamas.

I stewed in my misery. I had no other coping mechanisms than to sink into the darkness of being a victim once again, trapped in the body that I'd been in a fight with my whole life. The only solution left for my back was surgery.

I met with the neurosurgeon in August 2012 to discuss my options. He explained the severity of my rupture and its long-term effects, such as muscular imbalances, body compensation, and permanent nerve damage in my right leg. He recommended I have Microdiscectomy Spine Surgery.

Filled with incredible fear, I asked him a ton of questions. He had one question for me.

"How much longer do you want to live like this?"

"Not a second more," I answered.

I made the decision to have surgery.

After he explained the procedure, I felt confident in my decision. I now had something to look forward to—regaining my life. The following week, I arrived for surgery, and hours later, I walked out of the hospital standing up straight ... for the first time in months. When I arrived home, I asked Chuck if I could vacuum. I wanted to feel productive and contribute to having a normal life again. It was the best I'd felt in months, and I was ready to move on.

A few months later, I was able to start physical therapy. I worked out with a physical therapist, and it made me feel like I was back in the gym again. It gave me a feeling of accomplishment. *I can do this. After all, I am a bikini competitor,* I reminded myself. The staff didn't know I had lost. This could be a fresh start to prove myself.

One of the contributing factors in my extensive list of back issues was my weak posterior. I was underdeveloped, and my body over-compensated by using my lower back, which, given my pre-existing history, was at high risk.

No problem, nothing I can't fix. I'll figure it out when I'm cleared to lift again. I was determined—*until* the medical staff explained to me that I would never lift weights the way I did before. I had to avoid anything that would cause spinal compression, including movements such as forward flexion and running. Compound movements made up the majority of my lifts. They're what made me fall in love with lifting in the first place—the challenge, the progress, and the strength. It was all gone. No more. The end. I didn't have the insight to find other solutions or see that this was happening for me—to reshape my relationship with my body.

When you lose something you, you lose a part of our identity as well. You start asking yourself, *Who am I?*

I took on a new level of resentment and anger, starting with myself and continuing to those closest to me. Chuck felt

SEVEN

Silent Tears: Playing the Blame Game

In the days and weeks after the surgery, drugged up and lying in bed, I turned to social media. I followed fitness models and other bikini competitors as they prepared for Ms. Olympia and began living vicariously through their journeys. At first, my intention was to find inspiration. But after being told I'd never lift again, let alone compete, I looked at these perfect women as a reminder of what I'd never be. I felt the same comparison and jealousy that had been on rotation throughout my life.

On the outside, we lived a picture-perfect life filled with a happy marriage, vacations, and a thriving business, but in reality, it was a big mess. Something needed to change. My soul yearned for more. I tried different approaches—doing more, doing less, anything and everything—but I was still unhappy and stuck with an overwhelming feeling of sinking and struggling to survive. My physical limitations kept me confined to home most of the time, making me feel stagnant and resentful. Spiritually, I needed to grow.

I was looking to fill several missing aspects of my life and figured the best solution to this lack of growth was to go back to school and continue learning. I had to get back to basics and understand my spiritual foundation. I had to find God in all this mess.

In 2013, I expressed my lack of purpose and meaning to my younger brother John. He had started his own journey to personal development years earlier and had always been there to encourage me. I never actually got back to school, but the action of making a decision opened unexpected doors for me. I was repeating the cycle until John came down hard on me … no need to sugarcoat anything. We'd grown up learning to be assertive and direct, no excuses, only results. He told me, "We need to feel like we are contributing and growing constantly, or we lose our ability to thrive and live with purpose." This statement hit me hard. Purpose—that's what's missing!

I started writing again, which was something I did when I felt unseen or unheard. It was a release, but I hadn't written consistently since high school. Feeling rusty, and with so much to express, I started with a few sentences about how I felt, what I wanted to do, and what I wanted to accomplish. As I wrote my wants down, I realized they were all business-related. Having control over my business and seeing the results of my efforts allowed me to focus on the area I was good at—work. However, my work could only take me so far. My marriage and personal life were still in shambles.

I continued to pour my heart into my online business. It allowed me to continue to sit at home alone. I told myself, *If I could master my business, I'd be happy, and if I was happy, my marriage would be good.* If my marriage was good, we'd both have a happy, healthy, and wealthy home. Voila! The perfect formula—or so I thought. But man, how messed up is that?! How did I learn this way of thinking, rationalizing, and prioritizing beliefs? Were these even my own thoughts, or were they someone else's? Where were they learned? This piqued my curiosity, and I began to look back and ask questions.

Growing up, I didn't ask for help. I was strong, driven, and hustled to survive by stuffing my feelings down. I took pride in my work and rarely accepted credit for the success of my accomplishments. When life got hard, I didn't talk about it. What I felt, I pushed away. *Don't show signs of weakness—it'll be used against you.*

As the only girl, it was tough. I had to be tough. I didn't cry, show emotions, or talk about feelings. I believed they'd show my weakness.

Aside from my immediate family, I didn't talk to others about my problems. It was none of their business. They didn't need to know. *Be strong. Always strong.* Over the years, putting on this strong front and wearing a suit of armor got very heavy, and eventually, the armor began to crack.

When you survive by not showing signs of weakness, you learn to cry silently. You also lash out and fight back. You blame everyone for your problems and rationalize why your life sucks—*You don't understand.* I had all the excuses and reasons but could never admit my faults or flaws. I never took responsibility or ownership for the life I lived. It was always someone else's fault; they did me wrong.

In the process of shutting down emotionally, I never came to terms with my sexual abuse. Or maybe it was the abuse that had contributed to shutting me down.

When you're a little girl, and someone touches you inappropriately, you carry this feeling of shame with you for the rest of your life. I'd been resisting, dreading, and finding every way to avoid facing the reality of this incident.

Ironically, the fallout from the competition and the time spent facing my past forced me to start to love myself. Finally, I was able to express into words the emotions I felt about this experience. I could no longer downplay its impact on who I thought I was and what level of happiness I deserved.

The more I unraveled the abuse and researched its effects, the more I discovered how entwined it was with my body dysmorphia, eating disorders, anxiety, depression, obsessions, and addictions.

Finally Facing the Downside

I was in my early twenties when I first confided about the molestation to a friend, but I played it off nonchalantly. Some women had it way worse, and I felt what happened to me paled in comparison. It happened. It was a part of my story, and I didn't want to dwell on the past. I chose to keep moving forward while safeguarding my secret. Now I see that I was inherently crippled by that episode and would behave for most of my life in fight-or-flight mode.

At one point, I did confide in Jeremy. He wanted to take action against my abuser, but I wouldn't let him. In honor of my wishes, he took on the burden of my secret. Years later, I would mention the abuse in casual conversation with a few close girlfriends and wonder why it still bothered me. I told myself, *I'm over it, it was years ago,* but the damage was never repaired.

I was still suffering from the abuse and had no idea how deep the violation pierced. The truth is, there is no getting over sexual abuse until you face it and come to terms with it. It's not over, no matter what anyone says, until it is resolved personally and entirely for you. The incident became woven into the fabric of my life. It became a part of my story I didn't want to face.

Over the years, the more I shared my story, still playing it small and minimizing it, I saw how prevalent and normalized sexual abuse had become. Through sharing with other women, I realized I was not alone. Their innocence was stolen, and their lives forever changed. They also carried the scars. Many are too ashamed to speak out, too afraid of the judgment and condemnation that comes from others.

Because of how our culture is skewed—twisting scenarios, blaming the victims, making excuses, or pardoning the predators, it's hard for us women (and men) to speak about our abuse. And it's why we keep our secrets to ourselves, buried inside, festering like a cancerous sore until it becomes too big and, eventually, consumes us and those closest to us.

There is absolutely no justification for any act of sexual abuse.

A victim is a victim; there is no right or wrong. The perpetrator/predator knows exactly what their intentions are. Enough with the victim-blaming!

By remaining silent, we're discrediting our truth, a disservice to ourselves and others; this is not our secret to hold on to. Shame keeps us silent. We already feel *dirty* and worry about what others will think or say. We're made to feel as if it was our fault, that we deserved these inappropriate sexual acts as a form of punishment. By choosing to speak out, we're reopening the wounds, and for many, it's too painful to relive. We're all striving to do the best we can, and to heal and move on with our lives.

Little did I know that this one episode, this isolated incident, this breach of trust, would change the entire course of my life. The morning after the abuse, I had to face my abuser. I felt scared and powerless but had to pretend as if nothing had happened. Something shifted in me that morning. I felt violated all the way to my soul. It was then, looking at him and considering the number of lives it would affect if I chose to speak out. I shut down and kept my silence. In misguided altruism, I sacrificed my life to spare others. I created a mental and emotional prison for myself and lived within, serving a long-term sentence. In one unexplained moment as an innocent little girl, my life changed forever.

Throughout the years, I tried to downplay my incident. I carried shame, guilt, self-abuse, hurt, pain, and resentment for years. Layers upon layers of these negative emotions built up, and as time passed, I said, *What's the use? There's no reason to speak up now. It was years ago.*

I felt so ugly internally, as if, somehow, this was all my fault. I played what-if scenarios over and over again, trying to make sense of how and why this happened. *Why me?* Feeling so ashamed and dirty, the weight of carrying this secret around seeped into many areas of my life. I kept thinking something was wrong with me, like I was defective, disposable, and worthless garbage.

So much damage stemmed from this single violation that it warped my ability to trust, the perception of my own body, and how I treated myself *and* others. It colored how I looked at everyone and everything. I already knew and felt I was different before the abuse. It never occurred to me to look into the aftermath of sexual abuse and how its long-term effects played a significant part in my life. No longer was I willing to play the role of the victim, an *unfortunate child,* but that of a victor. I am a survivor.

The aftereffects wouldn't have made sense a few years ago when I was still trying to prove my worth on the stage. I wasn't at a place of self-awareness yet. I couldn't recognize the symptoms and hadn't learned what I know now. The cycle of guilt, shame, self-abuse, and self-loathing continued because I didn't have clarity about myself or my purpose.

I spent all these years torturing myself through various cycles of abuse and living in extremes from body dysmorphia to eating disorders, to self-esteem issues, to desperately trying to have a perfect body. My body was violated and felt damaged; I didn't want to live in this broken shell anymore. *If I perfected a new body,* I thought, *maybe I wouldn't have this film of shame over me.*

I was trying so hard to find my value and worth because my joy and innocence were stolen from me. The eating disorders (bingeing, starving, avoiding certain foods, taking laxatives, etc.) were ways I could control my body and how I looked and felt. I'd repeat the cycle over and over again, each time expecting different results.

In my mind and reflection in the mirror, I continued to see this overweight, ugly, and worthless person who no one wanted or loved, all the while chasing perfection. It was a self-imposed ideal.

I know now that perfection can never be met.

Now that I was coming to terms with the abuse, I was willing to change my thought process. But creating new thoughts and beliefs don't happen overnight. I had more time to spend in my funk before the mind shift took place. But it was knowing my younger brother was on my side that kept me hanging on. As I struggled to create new thinking habits, I managed to move only a few steps forward.

I found myself relapsing. I went back to my old ways of thinking. It's what I'd known my whole life. You don't know what you don't know, and it took a lot of practice, making mistakes, correcting, forgiving, and moving on. I had trust issues because I'd been burned way too many times. From early adolescence, my attitude and behavior changed after the abuse. While I began developing relationships, romantic and platonic, I struggled with opening up to trust and love. I never had a chance to understand and nurture love. I had mistaken love for niceness. If they didn't hurt me beyond my level of pain and abuse, this must be love.

The romantic relationships I had were awful. Prior to my husband, every guy I dated had cheated on me. But I was desperate to prove my worth and would beg them to take me back. I'd promise not to let them down again. *I can do better, be better. Let me be enough.* Looking back, I cry for the younger me. If only I'd had the courage to stand up for myself, then maybe I wouldn't have continued this abuse cycle for the majority of my life.

All I wanted was to be loved, but I didn't know or understand that. A person close to me, someone I was supposed to trust and love, had already violated that. So, what was love?

For my protection, I developed a hard exterior. Inside I was a broken little girl, emotionally damaged and weak. I was a little spitfire with a "don't mess with me" attitude. It was a defense mechanism (a shield I carried around at all times).

But at the same time, I was desperate. Inside I was begging, *Love me!*

I lived this mission of proving my self-worth throughout my life. It eventually led me to the stage for my first bikini competition. I'd show them I was good enough; I was of value. *I'm not this dirty, abused, disposable, or broken girl anymore. I've been through hell, and I'll show you, AND I won't even talk about it because we don't talk about this stuff.* I was willing to do anything for love and acceptance—except love and accept myself.

Until I could love myself, I wasn't able to develop a healthy, loving relationship with myself or others. The healing and journey to self-love involved many, many years of undoing the damage and rewiring my belief system. When I did finally start to love myself, the me I saw did not resemble the person willing to settle in my earlier years. I no longer needed to prove anything to anyone or to myself. As I grew into this new me, I accepted who and what I truly was.

The abuse part of my story had to be told in order for me to be free and live life as my best self: the fullest, most authentic representation of me. Determined to share my story, I let nothing hold me back from fulfilling my God-given purpose of inspiring, encouraging, and empowering others to live their best lives.

I was desperate for help and willing to do what it took to change my mindset. John, my younger brother, had become my biggest supporter. We were both dealing with the loss of Jeremy, so it made sense that we lean on each other for support A crisis can bring people together in a very profound way.

As I sat around, feeling sorry for myself, I asked, "Why me?" I tried praying and waiting. While I felt God had knocked me down for a reason, I wasn't happy about it.

He'd gotten me here, now what was His purpose and plan? Why was He doing this to me? What did I do wrong? I thought He wasn't showing up fast enough, so I tried to regain control, desperately grasping for anything to make it right. In my heightened state, I tuned in to every sound, listening for answers. But all I could hear was the sounds of my refrigerator going into defrost mode and some guy three doors down mowing his lawn. I was now outside myself on a whole new level.

The farther my life slipped away, the more desperate I became at gaining control. I had nothing left in me. My lack of understanding of love had been a factor in my marriage. I had been with my husband through everything, but not as the person I authentically wanted to be. When we change ourselves, it causes a ripple effect of unrest.

I blamed everyone for my problems: my husband, my trainer, my parents, my bad genes, and even God. Everyone was to blame—except me. I was drinking, raging, deflecting blame, and creating a toxic home environment. I had no idea I was hurting anyone, especially my husband. It was never my intention, but I hurt people as I was hurting.

This period in my life forced me to rethink how I was treating and talking to myself. No wonder I was a miserable person seeking validation on the stage and through others. How you speak to and treat yourself is a reflection of how you're accepting treatment from others. The amount of abuse we inflict on ourselves is the amount of abuse we're willing to accept from others. It's a validation of our self-worth.

I have one life, one body, one chance to be unique—to be me. Yet, I spent the majority of my life resenting, modifying, comparing, wishing to be anyone but me. This body was given to me as a vehicle to fulfill my purpose, to be the best version of myself. I wish I'd heard this message loud and clear a bit earlier—okay, much earlier!

Through all my pain and recovery, holed up in the house, it allowed me plenty of time to dwell on my past. I realized how my current and old thought patterns were no longer serving me.

As I started to seek a new path, I forced myself to create a gratitude journal. I still remember my first entry: I was grateful for myself. I wrote it down because I thought I was *supposed* to and wanted to see how it felt writing and saying it aloud.

I was grateful for my cat.

I was grateful for the weather.

It was a start.

What's one item you can write on a gratitude list today?

Points to Ponder

Do any of my behaviors sound familiar to you?

Do you exercise because it nurtures your body, or are you trying to prove something?

Do the people around you encourage and support you?

EIGHT

Inside the Tomb: Whoever Yells the Loudest Wins

My marriage hadn't been blessed with a great start. What should've been wedded bliss early on was torn apart by my brother's death, our attempts to start our own business together, the loss of my competition, and my back injury. We had a lot of challenges and complained about duties, finances—you name it, conflict consumed us.

I expected my husband to shoulder my emotional burden as I had no one else to turn to for support. I'd never confided in him about the abuse, and before I came to terms with it, I had no clue it was affecting our marriage. I had no clue it was affecting me. I wasn't processing the grief over my losses or my abuse with any form of therapy.

I was in a thick cloud of denial about everything. I felt broken and hurt everywhere. I had years of unhealed, deep wounds. Was my marriage headed down the crapper as a result?

Ironically, it was in my marriage that I felt significant, noticed, and controlling. It was a battleground for me. I got to assert the opinionated, bossy part of myself, the part that wasn't allowed to come out when I was a child. I lashed out, screamed, and yelled.

I poured my heart into our business, and the more effort I gave, the more my husband's contributions paled in comparison. Resentment started to build. I blamed and disliked him for not applying himself the way I did and felt he'd screw it up if I left anything unattended. I didn't trust him with the business when I couldn't be there to micromanage him. I wanted control. However, when it came to addressing the deep wounds in my personal life, I was thoroughly out of control.

Whoever yells the loudest wins. I always lost in life, but in this relationship, I won. I dominated by yelling, screaming, and belittling him. I needed to feel the power of control in a life that was spinning out of control. This storm of rage that had built up over time completely blindsided him. He tried to take it on, but I just pushed and pushed. Eventually, he learned to fight back using my tactics.

I couldn't believe this man stayed with me and still told me he loved me. *I'm not worthy of his love or anyone's love,* my mind told me. I couldn't and never did love myself. I questioned what love was. Why did love hurt so bad? How could someone love me? I'm broken and hard to love. I never felt beautiful, wanted, needed, or accepted. The more he tried, the more I pushed back. I absolutely loathed myself. I became a monster.

As I began to sink deeper into this abyss, I avoided reality by going out most nights and drinking. Alcohol helped take the edge off. Feeling frustrated and burned out, I'd finish work hungry and mentally drained. I just wanted to eat, relax, and go to bed. The problem was we didn't have meals prepared and were too tired to cook, so we'd go to a local restaurant for dinner and a drink.

We frequented one particular place so much that they'd pour our drinks as soon as we arrived and had them at the bar before we sat down. Some may call this excellent customer service, but I didn't like it. It was another form of unwanted negative attention. I didn't want to be noticed or remembered for my drinking or beverage choice. It embarrassed me. I expressed as much to my husband, "We need to find a new place—one where I can blend in with the crowd. I don't like this attention and don't want us to be known as *that drinking couple*. We're more than that."

However, our regular routines indicated otherwise. I'd order my usual Buffalo chicken wrap and onion rings, and a seasonal craft beer. I don't typically like beer. It makes me feel gassy and bloated, but this place wasn't exactly known for its wine or cocktail selection. I'd look over the beer list and choose based on which beer had the highest alcohol content. I was drinking only for the buzz.

After we placed our food order, I'd sit back and sip from the cute little snifter glass. The beer was always cold and refreshing. I'd stare at the TVs above the bar and mindlessly watch whatever sport was playing. I checked out. I didn't want to think or talk, just relax and give my overworked brain a rest. The beer went down smooth, and I'd order another. *It's only two beers,* I'd tell myself.

When the meal came, I dove into the Buffalo chicken wrap and onion rings doused in ketchup. I was so hungry! It hit the spot, and I'd feel another sensation of physical satisfaction. As the food settled, I'd feel sick from the grease and the heaviness of the meal. Immediately, guilt would overwhelm me. *Why hadn't I picked a better meal choice? Why do I continue to sabotage myself? Why did I eat this again?! Haven't I learned my lesson? I can't even run this off because of this stupid back injury ... wonderful!*

I had my gallbladder removed in 2006, but I could feel where it once fluttered in pain as my body tried to process a high-fat meal. I felt awful. I numbed my feelings with more alcohol. Now the acts of self-sabotage were replaced by self-loathing. With no answers found in this bar routine, I fell into a deep ditch. With my post-surgery back limitations, my diet was the one thing I had full control over. Yet I was ordering and devouring food like an uncontrollable, ravenous dog and feeling the pain and guilt of my poor choices. I was again losing control and punishing myself for it.

After dinner and a few drinks, we had no desire to head home. Any place was better than home. Our home had become a tomb. We did whatever it took to avoid and not deal with it. We didn't confront our issues with real conversations—I didn't know how. When my husband wanted to talk, I'd dismiss him. I could feel my heart race with anxiety and panic at the mention of the words, "We need to talk." Immediately, I shifted into defense mode, plotting how I could I turn it on him and protect myself. *No, we don't need to talk. I'll tell you how it is.* Engaging in actual dialogue made me way too uncomfortable. We made efforts to connect, but we were speaking two different languages. He had conversation and communication. I, on the other hand, had yelling and demanding. As you can imagine, that got us nowhere.

My social environment was the bars. I could be anonymous and not share anything about myself. I could get to know fellow bar-goers on a superficial level through drinking, shallow conversation, and watching sports on TV. It was a perfect place to hide from any problems at home and within myself.

I would sit on my barstool and watch some old guy make a complete mess of himself. I would think, *Are you kidding me? At least I am not that guy.* Yes, without a trace of irony, I would consider myself lucky not to be *that* drunk at the bar. But how much better off was I?

Some nights, we needed more than one bar. I would connect with women and laugh, and he would talk with the guys about sports and whatnot. I felt the effects of the alcohol and felt uninhibited. Getting drunk allowed me to be someone else. I connected and talked to anyone—the complete opposite of who I am without alcohol. When drunk, I was no longer quiet and reserved, and I didn't wait to be spoken to before I spoke up.

At home, we'd spend hours arguing back and forth with offensive name-calling and accusations. We both hurt so deep inside but couldn't—and didn't—know how to communicate with each other. Yelling and screaming were our forms of communication. This vicious cycle of verbal abuse was the norm; it was all I knew. We'd argue and fight almost every night and wake up resenting each other. Our drunken fights blurred into the next day and eventually became our new life.

One of our newly coupled friends told my husband, "You two have the perfect marriage. It's what I want for us."

I literally laughed out loud when my husband mentioned this. I said, "We're that good, huh?" We'd been playing this *perfect life* role all too well. We even had our friends and family fooled. How little did they know?

Most evenings, I went out and looked forward to the excitement and the new connections I'd make—two needs I lacked at home and sought elsewhere. We had a structured nightly schedule and made sure we could keep a sense of anonymity by rotating to different drinking establishments. I didn't want people to know me. I could hide among the crowd. In all these places, people were numbing their pain. We were two of them.

I was ashamed of what I'd become. This felt like a huge step backward. I fought long and hard to escape these places of self-commiseration. This was me many years ago. It felt wrong in so many ways, but I had no other option. I had given up life as I knew it and wasn't on any spiritual journey yet.

Other than drinking to escape and numb our pain, I had nothing in common with these strangers. The intrigue and mystery of who we would meet on any given night kept the excitement alive. These connections made for good company during the dark times until I no longer needed them. I knew I wouldn't have to see those strangers again (unless they too were on the same rotating bar schedule). I got what I came for: *get in, get numb, get out, move on, and forget.*

Eventually, I realized that what I was doing was wrong. Even though I was struggling to find who I was, I knew this wasn't me. I wasn't growing; I was still playing small, stuck in the darkness. I was retreating to the loneliness of a bar to drink my miserable life away. Or at the least, numb myself and not remember it.

So why was I there? I didn't understand at the time that my soul-searching required this view of my life so I could see people behaving in this way. I needed it for perspective as I sought a brighter path. I knew one day, I could inspire people ready to take a different course of action in their lives. If we don't have the darkness, we can't speak about how we found the light.

As the evening turned to night, we'd come home drunk, feeling the liquid courage and vulnerability. We tried to continue having the same fun and exciting connection amongst ourselves. But that didn't work. Our conversations quickly escalated and turned into an explosive verbal war. It would start by one of us making a snide comment, and that's all the spark that was needed. The battle began. I'd call him a loser and tell him he was wasting my time and money. I was working twice as hard to support this household and live this *perfect* lifestyle of doing what we want when we want. I told him he was a freeloader and a trophy husband. I felt used, abused, and taken for granted. He'd fight back, telling me how everyone thought I was pretentious, shallow, and worthless.

Initially, we attended marriage counseling, but I didn't realize how messed up *I* was until I started seeing the counselor on my own. I had years' worth of baggage to unpack. I told the counselor about the abuse and played it off as no big deal. He suggested I tell my husband.

I was afraid Chuck might reject me. So, I gave him a watered-down version. That was his first time hearing about it. A year later, as we were planning a trip to Thailand, my counselor advised me to tell Chuck the whole story before the vacation, and so I did. I told Chuck the truth.

I'd been withholding so much from him and missing out on having a passionate and intimate relationship. That kind of relationship was something I'd longed for but never knew or understood. I was afraid of what Chuck would think and how he would see me. I was afraid of being hurt again by allowing him to know my deep dark secret. I was scared he'd leave me and reject me like all the previous boyfriends had. All the fighting, screaming, heated arguments were really a cry for help from a wounded soul. When I told my husband about the abuse, it shocked him. Immediately, he wanted to confront the guy and defend me. That didn't matter anymore to me. I was so relieved he now knew. Now that I'd told my husband about the abuse and had gotten off the barstool, I turned my focus back to the demons of fitness.

You can't move on from fitness until you've resolved fitness, especially since I'd been battling it my whole life. Likewise, you can't move on from abuse until you've talked about abuse. The same applies to any area in your life causing the most resistance. Trying to outrun, numb, or find solace in other forms is only preventing the wounds from healing. Let's acknowledge, heal, and move forward.

Even if your life feels inherently messed up, know it's not your fault. There's no point in spending any more time beating yourself up about the past. What is done is done. It's only your fault if you choose to stay messed up and be in denial. You need to get out of your own way and make a change *now*.

My *now* had to be one step at a time and involved a lot of new questions. There is so much more to life than blame, misery, loneliness, guilt, shame, and abuse. You are in control of your life, whether it feels like it or not, but everything you do is a choice made by you. I made the first choice to wonder and ask, *Could I live my life in a different way?*

Points to Ponder

Take a look at your current social situation.

Are you hanging in social circles that don't serve you and exist solely to let you hide from your inner demons?

In what ways is it growing and enriching your life?

What are some ways it confines and limits you?

In what ways are you willing to step outside your comfort zone?

You need to get comfortable with being uncomfortable and be honest with yourself.

You are the average of the five people you spend
the most time with.
—Jim Rohn

Change happens when the pain of staying the same
is greater than the pain of change.
—Tony Robbins

NINE

I Don't Have Time: When the Student Is Ready

The physical limitations and restrictions that accompanied my back injury also brought me back to the subject of diet and nutrition. I wanted to know how the female competitors maintained their physiques in the off-season. There had to be an alternative to eating the same boring foods. That's not living! Determined to find a solution to living with balance, moderation, and enjoyment, I saw these women as beacons of hope. I knew there was an alternate way; I just needed to find it. I didn't know at the time that I'd take the stage again in a bikini competition. Or that I was working toward a new mode of performing—one rooted in a place of self-acceptance and self-love, a new life.

The Eating Trap

Everything seemed to be on one extreme diet or another of *healthy* or *clean* eating. Information overload from these various fads and diets quickly overwhelmed me. The "noise" grew louder and louder. Where was I supposed to begin?

During my first competition prep, the belief was that you had to follow a rigid and strict diet of *clean* foods such as chicken, broccoli, and rice. It was the old-school bodybuilding mentality, and apparently, that's how you won competitions. Food and labels only added to my confusion. It led to another belief that if I strayed from *clean eating,* then it must mean the food I ate was *dirty.* Therefore, I was dirty. *You are what you eat,* right? This belief birthed new fears and anxieties, which, in turn, led to another eating disorder. Like I needed something else wrong with me.

There had been little talk of what life would be like post-competition, just the mention of "you can't go back to eating how you did before." *Okay, thanks!* Where is this gray area called balance and moderation? Unfortunately, it wasn't explained or taught in a way that made sense to me. I'd been on an extreme diet to get my body stage-ready for the competition and hoped the *extreme* would be worth it. What I *really* wanted was a quick fix to liking myself, hoping to undo the years of self-loathing and self-abuse.

After the competition, I was mentally, physically, and emotionally destroyed. I didn't know what to think, let alone how to create a new lifestyle. Nothing was in my favor at this point as I continued being miserable and confused by this diet mystery and riddle.

In my old extreme and rigid mindset, I believed that eating *dirty* or *bad* foods would erase the progress I'd made. I would feel guilty for making *poor* choices and try to make up for them by using exercise as a form of punishment—especially running—defining my unending cycle of abuse, punish, repeat.

Discovering Flexible Dieting

After years of misleading information and limited science and education in the diet and fitness world, it was my brother John, who introduced me to Flexible Dieting. Flexible Dieting is a lifestyle that follows the belief that no foods are off-limits. There are no foods that are inherently good or bad—food is food. All foods have calories and macronutrients. There are three macronutrients: proteins, fats (lipids), and carbohydrates (sugar). Each macronutrient provides energy in the form of calories. We need calories to survive and thrive; they're essential to our overall health and well-being. Flexible Dieting provides structure and balance to ensure your body gets the proper nutrition and fuel required to function while achieving a desired body composition goal. Whether your goal is losing fat, gaining lean muscle, or improving your overall performance, consuming the proper amount of macronutrients is key.

Finally, a diet that's evidence and science-based with numerous case studies to back it up. I now had some insight into how this diet mystery and riddle could be solved for me!

Flexible Dieting teaches you what to eat and how to eat, allowing you to ditch the diet mentality and break free of the antiquated methods of restrictive, extreme diets and eliminating the yo-yo diet cycle. No more meal plans, no more fads, and no more gimmicks.

I made a commitment to a lifestyle change, starting with diet and nutrition. It challenged me at first, but with my brother's support, I shifted my focus from what I didn't want to what I did want—food freedom. Having trust issues because of the many failed attempts in the past at this whole dieting thing, I was skeptical at first. I began educating myself. Along with John's help, I learned how to calculate my calories and macronutrients (macros) and began creating and living a lifestyle of food freedom.

Although I now knew how to count, track, and *budget* my macros, I wasn't fully confident about lifting weights again. The doctors cleared me to resume light activity, however, I was still overprotective and afraid of re-injuring my back. After much debate and excuse after excuse, my brother John convinced me to conquer my fears and start lifting weights again. He offered to write a basic strength training program and encouraged me to start with the basics: bodyweight.

After years of not lifting and overcoming my injury, I was afraid to see how much strength I'd lost. However, this allowed me a neutral foundation to build upon. Starting fresh with a new training plan, I was just grateful to be able to move!

Feeling overwhelmed by the information and videos found on YouTube and social media, I was fortunate to have a workout plan to go with my food macros. I jumped in with both feet, but immediately, I felt the fear and resistance like many people do when first starting. It scared me. I judged myself according to my old pattern and fell into the mindset of limiting beliefs and excuses. I was in denial. I would tell myself that I don't know what I'm doing. *I shouldn't be here. I'm not ready. I don't have time. This is not a priority.* What I really meant was *I am not a priority.*

Feeling pressed for time, I half-assed the workouts, and on some days, I wouldn't make it to the gym at all. I would blame my half-heartedness on my busy life and schedule; when the truth was, I felt stuck. I needed help, but I didn't believe

I deserved it. I launched a new lifestyle but was still running a solo show. I didn't know how to trust or ask for support.

"I don't have time" is a lame excuse! We all have the same amount of time. It's just a matter of how we choose to spend it and how we manage our priorities. Watch how quickly plans change and our schedules adjust. Suddenly, we're able to fit in life events and distractions that just pop up, like happy hours, lunch dates, and shopping. As plans change, your goal should stay the same. By saying yes to everyone and everything else, we end up saying no to ourselves, and we resist the opportunity to become a priority.

By not making my health a major priority, I fed into the stories, lies, and excuses I'd been telling myself. It gave me the attention I needed without even trying. My problems and reasons were no different than those of others; it gave me a sense of camaraderie with other women like me. We'd sit, stew, and play the "I don't have time" game. I had a different excuse depending on the company and my mood at the time.

As a self-proclaimed professional multi-tasker, I added fitness to my fully stacked plate, thinking it was just one more thing I could accomplish. However, this being the newest and lowest on the priority list, I neglected it. I thought I'd just figure it out on my own, like I always did.

After a few months of repeatedly half-hearting my efforts, I couldn't understand why I wasn't making any progress. I took monthly progress pictures, measurements, and weighed myself, yet nothing had changed. My weight and fitness levels were the same because I wasn't one hundred percent committed. I hadn't changed anything other than the idea of wanting change. I knew I wanted something different.

Accepting the Idea of a Mentor

At this point, John was still my primary support. He mentioned how hiring a coach had helped him with creating structure, planning, learning, and understanding, and he suggested I do the same. I'd been following fitness coach, Sohee Lee[6], online and loved her philosophy and approach to diet and nutrition. She was uniquely relatable. I hadn't found this with other coaches. I connected to her story and her struggles with extremes such as yo-yo dieting, binging, excessive cardio, and the strive for the perfect body mentality. She and I shared similarities that were unique to our stories, and I was in awe at how she overcame them. I, too, wanted to overcome my struggles and find a balanced and healthy approach to fitness and nutrition.

I mentioned her to my brother, and his coach, Layne Norton, highly recommended her and thought she'd be a perfect fit for me. Everyone was giving me the go-ahead. *Could I do it?*

The excuses kicked in. This online coaching thing made little sense to me. *Didn't they need to see me? How were they going to help me if they didn't know me? What was this whole virtual thing, anyway? And the cost?! How could I even know if I was coachable? Besides, who was this woman, anyway? How and why would I pay for someone I didn't know and would most likely fail me?* I didn't trust anyone. *I* was too much work. To my surprise, John met my excuses with an offer to help. I was shocked! He saw potential in me when I didn't and was willing to invest in it … in me. Sometimes, the people in your life are there to show you that you're worth it when you've lost all belief in yourself.

I assumed that mentors were people who didn't struggle, that their lives were easy, and they made a killing charging others to help them figure out their lives or how to make it as big as they did. I was so wrong!

Mentors aren't necessarily found outside of a core support circle. They can simply be a family member, friend, coach, or teacher. If these examples don't apply to you, don't give up. Don't stop looking in your current community. Don't give up looking for support at any point. We all need it and should receive it with gratitude. It's okay to ask for help. It's not a sign of weakness. Rather, it's a sign of strength and courage. Ask, and you shall receive.

I have a few suggestions if you're struggling with body image, fitness, nutrition, and overall self-love:

- Talk to a family member, friend, coach, or teacher.
- Find a mentor.
- Ask a staff member at the gym to show you how to use the equipment.
- Seek professional help (counselors, therapists, doctors, dietitians, or a nutritionist).
- Find like-minded community groups, for example, at your local church, gym, or neighborhood. You can find groups to join or host on Meetup.com, and of course, Facebook has groups for everything!

A mentor is a trusted person you admire and respect and someone who has your best interests at heart. Mentorship is a relationship between a more experienced or more knowledgeable person (a teacher) and a person with less experience or less knowledge (a student).

My brother's compassion and grasp of where I was, where I was heading, and knowing I needed help was a turning point in my life. I hadn't realized it at the time, but my brother had become my first mentor.

I gratefully accepted John's offer to meet me halfway with hiring Sohee, and we set the ball in motion. I committed myself to not letting him down and also to not letting my new coach down. Having this type of accountability and commitment, both monetary and personal, was exactly what I needed.

Little did I know that by trusting Sohee, it would also help me in trusting other key people in my life, some of whom I would work with later.

Getting to Know Sohee

Sohee's evidence-based approach to fitness and nutrition is one that uses sustainable and enjoyable methods for creating lifelong fitness. She'd struggled with eating disorders and body image, and she was also a bikini competitor. I felt as though she understood me, not because of our shared struggles but because of the actions she took to overcome them. She was proof of change and a beacon of hope.

I wanted to overcome my struggles. After all these years, barely staying afloat, I committed to changing my life. In September 2014, I took that leap of faith and hired Sohee for one-on-one training and nutrition coaching. I hired her for a three-month period—short enough to ease my insecurities but long enough to know if I would see changes. In three months, I would know if my decision had been beneficial and a good fit between student and teacher.

Adjusting to the mentality of being accountable wasn't easy at first. I made a ton of mistakes. Many days, I fell short of my targeted macros because I was afraid to overeat. I thought if I just ate less, it'd work in my favor. Calories in versus calories out, right? *Nope.* It wasn't that simple, or I wouldn't have needed Sohee's help. She encouraged me to continue trusting her and to trust the process. It was okay to eat more—my body needed it.

In the beginning, while still working out the kinks, I learned which foods to *spend* my macro budget on. I often made poor and expensive food choices, costing me my macros and left me hungry and heading to bed early to start over the next day. I'd extend myself grace and used these mistakes as learning curves.

I began to look at food and its nutritional value through a new lens as I swapped my *expensive* foods with *more affordable* options. For example, I'd trade a big bowl of Cocoa Pebbles for a giant, colorful salad topped with lean meat and a glass of red wine. Sure, the bowl of cereal sounded like a delicious choice, but it had little to no nutritional value and left me feeling hungry shortly afterward. On the flip side, the giant, nutrient-dense salad with lean meat took forever to eat and left me feeling full and satisfied. And as an added perk, a glass of wine. I set myself up to win and rewarded my new behavior choices with treats I enjoyed. Quickly, I learned to spend my macros wisely and how to get more bang for my *macro buck.*

When I committed fully to changing my life, I hired mentors and coaches for help in other areas of my personal and professional life. It was the start I needed. They inspired and encouraged me to create the life I wanted. A few of the influencers, mentors, coaches, and authors that hugely impacted my life are Tony Robbins, Sohee Lee, Brené Brown, Ruby Fremon, and Kim O'Hara.

Scared from my previous letdowns and uncertainties, I had no choice but to keep an open mind. Slow healing occurred through prayer, meditation, fitness, and writing. I decided to squeeze every last cent out of this investment to change and learn as much as possible. For when the student is ready, the teacher appears. I was ready.

Points to Ponder

What is your opinion of having a mentor?

What are your relationships with time, health, and fitness?

In what ways do you treat your body with love and respect?

What is your favorite excuse for not seeking support?

The significant problems we face cannot be solved at the same level of thinking we were at when we created them.
—Albert Einstein

TEN

Gymtimidation: As Real as a Stepford Wife

I learned, through trial and error, to listen to trusted people when they offer advice and support. Sometimes this is not an accident but a divine intervention. If you've tried to exert control over your life and reaped plenty of mistakes, perhaps it's time to be open to advice from those who've gone before you and want the best for you.

Over the first three weeks of working with Sohee, my desire to quit was fueled by the limiting belief that I couldn't do this. Easing out of my comfort zone was tough, and at times, I asked myself, *What's the point?* But determined to stay the course and not disappoint my coach, I gave it my all. I eventually started to see small changes in my body, strength training, and nutrition. I used the progress as momentum to keep moving forward and a reminder that I was on the right track.

Many days, I exceeded my macros resulting in overeating. I feared that I would somehow regress and negate any progress

I'd made. This gave me anxiety, leading me down the *I'm a failure* path. Learning this new lifestyle took practice, time, and overcoming frustration. Sohee kept me motivated through our daily and weekly communications, which were necessary and thorough. I embraced her accountability and encouragement. She supported me with questions, "How do you look?" and "How do you feel?" Sohee developed personal training programs specifically designed to work around my physical limitations (avoiding spinal compression and flexion) and focused on strengthening my posterior.

At first, admittedly, I had my guard up and was afraid to be vulnerable and transparent. I would answer her questions with vague responses. I'd been burned far too many times by being naive, exposed, and honest. Since she and the process were new, they both had to earn my trust. I carried with me the unease and trust issues from previous relationships and past personal trainers—let alone my pre-existing physical conditions.

What if I fail? What if I get hurt again? These types of fears were crippling, not just in the fitness aspect, but in my attitude towards life overall. Fear held me back. I thought I was a loser. I was too scared to let go. With my need for control, no wonder I landed at the bottom.

All dressed up and armed with my water bottle and training program, I walked into the gym with my head up, ready to take on the world. Then I looked around. Reality and *gymtimidation* set in—the bright lights, noises, people, and the clanking of weights overwhelmed me. I retreated within, and once again, fear reared its ugly head.

Heading into the gym solo triggered memories of my numerous failed attempts. I felt the familiarity creeping in, and it tempted me to avoid the machines and stick to cardio. Even though I had a plan, I still felt intimidated and clueless.

A lot of the exercises on Sohee's training plan were unfamiliar or weird looking, like frog pumps and hip thrusts. I had never seen them done before, which led to a good part of my time spent in the corner of the gym, looking up videos on YouTube. I tried to replicate them without drawing attention to myself. I avoided all eye contact and did my best to stay out of people's way. I just wanted to get in, get out, and move on with my day.

While working through the fears of re-injuring my back, I executed the prescribed training programs. The program's design was to focus on progressive overload—progressively doing more while getting stronger over time. Starting at the bottom again, slowly but surely, I advanced from bodyweight to dumbbells, to barbells, and eventually, to loaded barbells. I'd gone my entire life forcing outcomes by sheer will and feeling little to no joy in the process. How could one have joy when expecting failure?

With my marriage on standby, I worked on what I could control. Chuck felt rejected, knowing I'd hired a coach online to train me when he had a degree in sports and exercise studies. At this time, we were still codependent and fractured. Fitness coaching lessened the desire to take my frustrations out on him. Instead of falling back into my old ways of attacking verbally, I filled myself in a new way—with spirituality.

A friend invited me to a women's retreat called *Prosper* through a local church, and I saw a new path opening. My only prior exposure to faith-based events, primarily among women, had been what I'd seen on TV. I attended the event claiming to have an open mind, but honestly, I thought it would be one of those stiff Christian gigs where the ladies would be on their best behavior—prim, proper, and perfect. I envisioned a Christian version of *The Stepford Wives*[7], all secretly judging and keeping tally. Oh, I was so wrong. The only one judging was me! You see, once again, I'd fallen for the media stereotypes. This time, of what a Christian's *supposed* to be, primarily a Christian woman. Although I shared the Christian faith, mine was weak.

The women were welcoming, warm, and kind, and they shared their pains, struggles, and prayers with the group. Once there, still new to networking and socializing, I lowered my guard, thinking, *Ah, these women aren't so bad.* We did a few arts and crafts projects for the homeless and hospitals. Volunteering and creativity are both passions of mine, and I soon found myself settling in. The women even showed an interest in me and asked questions. They genuinely wanted to know me. They provided community and connection. I didn't realize it at the time, but community was something I lacked. I wanted to fit in and belong, quite the opposite of all my preconceptions.

Surrounded by the community, it was an honor and a blessing that they accepted and let me in. They were far from the perfect women I'd expected them to be. We're all flawed, perfectly imperfect, doing our best to honor and serve a perfect God. I decided I would give this faith thing a try. I tried it on, it felt good, and the next morning, I attended my first church service.

Once I was ready to accept change, God began to do His work on me and through me, letting me know I wasn't alone. After a few months, Chuck began to see a change, and he, too, started to attend service with me. We've been going ever since.

Points to Ponder

How often do you worry about what others think?

In what areas of your life do you doubt yourself?

In what areas do you lack trust and confidence in your abilities?

What is a spirituality belief that's unique to you?

Where can you seek a spiritual community?

ELEVEN

The Gift of Inspiration: Accepting Humility and Confidence

Having a coach and hearing words of encouragement helped build my confidence. Sohee provided constructive feedback from the videos and pictures I'd send her. "I don't know what the hell I'm doing," I wrote to her. She would reply with positive messages combined with a few adjustments to how I was thinking and speaking about my body.

Sohee helped reframe my thinking from negative to positive. When I couldn't or wouldn't see my own progress, she would remind me of the inches I'd lost. She helped me *see* my results. That kept me motivated and focused on the big picture.

One day, I had an *Oh, I got this* moment. While performing one of those weird exercises—hip thrusts—I saw a girl sitting in the corner, facing my direction with a phone in her lap. I smiled at her as my immediate thought was, *that was me back when I first started—confused and scared, sitting in the gym corner, looking up videos on YouTube.* Then, it hit me! She wasn't looking up videos; she was recording me! My perception shifted.

People were no longer looking at me because I was clueless. They were looking at me because I knew what I was doing, and I saw how that was inspiring others. I finally owned my history in a positive way. When she saw me smile in her camera, she knew she was caught and was embarrassed. I gave her another smile as I finished my set and moved on. I didn't want her to feel uncomfortable.

A short time later, I passed her again, only this time she was attempting to do the same movement, a hip thrust. I stopped to help her with set up and offered to let her use my hip pad for the bar. She thanked me and was grateful for my help.

Another day, a well-built guy approached me. I tend to keep to myself at the gym, as it's a form of therapy. I go there to be alone inside my mind while working on my body. I'm fully aware of my surroundings and ready to offer help or share my passion for training and nutrition. Shoptalk is enjoyable with other women as we share common interests. But when this big dude approached me, it caught me off guard. "Seeing you in the gym lifting is inspiring," he said. "You are one of the strongest and smallest people I know, and I heard you had back surgery too."

"Thanks!" I said. He admitted he had similar back issues and was also considering surgery. I shared with him the process and steps I took: injections, physical therapy, and the pain meds all before I had surgery. I'm not a doctor but was happy to share my personal experiences. I suggested he consult his doctor to determine what might work best for him.

He was also the first person to bring to my attention that other people regarded me as an inspiration. I found this kind of creepy at first. I didn't want the attention, but through my personal growth, I graciously took the compliment and learned to accept it.

I hadn't considered that I was an inspiration, even though people were showing up now to tell me. It made me feel something I'd never felt—fulfilled and purposeful. As I shared parts of my story, it began to resonate with others, and I realized I was not alone. I didn't have to go through the pain for nothing. There was a point after all; I could help people who were still suffering, a few years behind me in their progress—or more. I had an inkling that I would soon be living my purpose of helping others and tapping into one of my gifts—inspiration.

If you're inspiring others, you also begin to have love and compassion for yourself. You recognize that you're contributing good in the world. The more you are serving others and using your past struggles as gifts in the present, the more fulfilled you become. Regardless of whether I felt I deserved compliments or kind words, I knew my perspective had shifted. It wasn't about them complimenting me. It was about me inspiring them.

I still smile today as I recall one of the best compliments I have ever received. I was setting up for an incline bench press when one of the trainers, also a bodybuilder and competitor, was talking with a new gym employee, and they walked toward me. I began to take out my earbuds. "Hey," he said. "No need for that, I'm just here to talk you up." I gave him a confused look as he introduced me to the new girl as, "One of the most inspiring women at the gym." My jaw dropped; I was dumbfounded. He continued, but I was still caught on his first line. *Was he really talking about me?!*

He continued with more compliments, building me up in front of someone I'd never met before. After the slew of praises, still smiling, I introduced myself to her. Those were the only words I could utter. Wow, just wow! I was on cloud nine for the rest of the day. I didn't know what to say. This had never happened to me, and it took me a day to process my thoughts and feelings. I didn't know then how to respond with gratitude and humility—how to accept compliments graciously, but I do now. There was no need for awe or silence. I admitted to myself, I could be an example, to inspire, and to help others.

The next day, I thanked him from a place deep in my heart. "No one's ever spoken so highly of me," I told him. "That meant a lot." I told him I had no idea what others thought of me at the gym. But then again, it didn't matter what they thought. I came to the gym to *do me*.

"By living and doing you, that is humbling, and others take notice," he said.

"Thank you." I simply replied.

A smile emerged as I recalled the mantra I had created for myself. I looked at my bracelet and read the inscription: Inspire. Encourage. Empower.

Sohee's Program Continues

In the beginning, I was wary and kept my victim mentality—I thought it was still serving and protecting me. I wanted the lifestyle and transformation process to happen as quickly and painlessly as possible.

On one of my bi-weekly check-ins, Sohee asked me, "What do you see in the mirror?"

"I see the same shape and image every time I look in the mirror," I responded. "I am feeling very soft and fluffy around my midsection and love handle area. My legs look bigger but stronger."

Sohee was kind and thoughtful as she answered, "The progress is slow, but it's definitely there. You lost half an inch off your waist, and that's nothing to scoff at. As long as you continue to train hard and nail your nutrition, you'll also notice a gradual shift in body composition over time."

Through her patient and encouraging coaching style, I began seeing results in her program. I built trust. Having a support system was new and felt amazing. Someone was rooting for me! I was also inspiring others at the gym, which made a huge difference for me.

Progressing each week on my training, I felt strong, empowered, and that something new was taking place in me. It felt weird. I didn't know what to make of it. This feeling was confidence—something I longed for and admired in others. I not only built upon this new foundation of confidence, but it also became a big, mental middle-finger to all those who I felt had limited me. Crushing my workouts and having someone believe in me caused my life to take a different shape. I was curious about my new direction and potential and surprised myself by how open I was to the unknown. Having potential and confidence in myself allowed me to see the daily progress outside of the gym, in the mirror, in myself, and in life.

I rejected negative mindsets and those who existed in my social life up to this point. I was on a quest to surround myself with like-minded people, ready and willing to level up and invest in themselves personally and professionally. I wanted to keep the momentum moving, looking forward and upward.

I was looking at everything with fresh eyes and, for the first time, content and genuinely happy. A new feeling came from a place I'd never known. *Was this real life?*

Previously, I searched for answers externally, and now I'd created this small change from within. To understand it was there this whole time, inside me, was incredible. I lived most of my life in extremes: all-or-nothing, black-and-white, always-or-never.

Taking on a new mindset was hard. Living in extremes had become easy. In embracing the process of letting go, I allowed my old ways of extreme thinking to fade. I leaned into a new and wiser approach, one of balance and moderation. The experience was a high I'd never known, and it became addicting.

And I created another mantra:

Consistency compounded over time yields results.

Wow! Who is this girl?

Redefining Failure

I also had to redefine failure. I would no longer say, "I am a failure." From that point on, if I fail at something, it's called a lesson. I learned from what didn't work and take the opportunity to try again and keep growing. Fitness was once something I did to look and feel like my perception of perfection, no matter its cost to my mental, emotional, and physical health.

But now I was living for me and for all the right reasons. I had the right mindset and the right coach. There would no longer be any overtaxing, binging, starving, overeating, or mistreating myself to radical extremes. No more gimmicks, pills, or supplements, which claimed that if I took two pills before a greasy meal, it would magically rid the meal of all the fat. I decided I could have clarity, confidence, joy, and success with fitness and still be passionate about it.

I understood this was a maintenance program of confidence. Building confidence allowed me to develop and strengthen my body for reasons other than health and fitness. It allowed me the foundation to grow in all other areas of my life, like love and career, while taking on this new mindset and sense of self. Where I was lost, I had to be found.

My mindset shifted, and a glimmer of self-love and self-confidence began to blossom within the short three-month period of working with Sohee. I needed this shift since I was a child. When our initial three months were up, I wanted to test my new self by navigating the holiday season without any coaching guidance. This would be the *road test* of what I'd learned to see if I could survive on my own with the tools and resources Sohee had imparted.

My first holiday alone with no coaching or anyone to hold my hand was a success! I was anxiety-free! For the first time in years, I spent more time enjoying the holidays than I did worrying and stressing over food, my body, or the damn scale. Holiday dinners and desserts were non-issues. I didn't need to weigh and track my food, and I didn't rebound in gaining back the little bit of weight I'd lost. I felt confident in myself and my flexible dieting skills.

At this time, Sohee had just finished a bikini competition of her own. I asked her about her competition experience, and she explained that her approach was to use the same philosophy and tools she preached and taught to others. I admitted I was still longing to compete again as a different person. She agreed, suggesting that it would be transformative and healing to compete in another show. That first competition experience couldn't be the end of my fitness story.

A month after the holidays, I hired Sohee back on. I wanted to compete again. This time it would be different, completely different. I was different.

Points to Ponder

How do you define *failure?*

Which areas of your life do you consider a failure?

How could you find joy, a blessing, or a lesson somewhere in that area?

Do you think you deserve joy? If not, why?

Can you create a new mantra for yourself today?

TWELVE

Finding Freedom: Surrender to Self

Contemplating another competition would be a night and day difference. I couldn't let my first bodybuilding competition in 2012 be my last. I would try again, but this time with an entirely new approach, new coach, new plan, new mindset, new person, and a new suit. New everything! I was excited and looked forward to it. This year, 2015, was my year of redemption. Everything I did wrong the first time, I wanted to do right.

When I first started lifting weights with my coach's guidance, the insecurity about my legs—that old childhood complex—reared up again. Sometimes our egos will do whatever it takes to stop us in our tracks when we're venturing into a brave new direction. I feared my legs would get bigger. I fell victim to that gym myth that lifting weights would make me bulky, and I tried to avoid anything that would make my legs bigger and more noticeable. However, when I started training for the first 2015 fitness competition, I had to get over that fear quickly. Lifting weights did not make me big nor bulky but gave me a toned definition and shape, exactly what I was looking to achieve. I continued to make progress and set personal records—which Sohee and I call PRs—impressing both myself and others.

I forced myself, as uncomfortable as it was, to embrace my body and legs, flaws, and all. What changed the most was my mindset and how I viewed my body. I could finally make sense of that girl's comment made back in 2012 about my legs. She had honestly, without any ill will, truly admired them.

Today, I am thankful for the strength of my legs, and most of all, grateful that I have them! When it comes down to it, what we hate about ourselves can be loved when we are grateful for what we have.

I began to build strength and confidence through my newfound love and passion, strength training. My thick, solid, huge, *ugly* legs now had a place and a purpose in the gym. They became my greatest asset and tool. I learned to embrace the process of building my legs to improve my workouts and prevent further injury to myself.

I noticed other women training so hard to get big, thick legs while I had dressed mine in any way possible to hide them. I'd taken them for granted. What I'd resented, I found others desiring!

I started to take notice of what others perceived as flaws and found myself admiring and nurturing the same qualities in myself. When we're too focused on our egos and our imperfections, we lose sight and forget that we have everything we need inside.

Throughout my entire contest prep, I practiced Flexible Dieting and used the *no foods off-limits* approach. Never once did I feel deprived or guilty; never once did I starve or binge as I had in 2012. I took an 80/20 approach to eating whole, healthy, real foods. Eighty percent went to nutrition while the remaining twenty percent were for treats, if I desired, as long as they fit my macros. For example, my diet primarily consisted of lean meats, veggies, and complex carbs while saving room for a sweet treat, like chocolate, desserts, or an occasional glass of wine, if I could fit them into that day.

My coach continued to adjust my macros as needed. Because I'm petite and cutting more calories would be counterproductive, Sohee adjusted my exercise to sprinkle in cardio and High Intensity Interval Training (HIIT), as needed.

There was no reason to overdo anything, no more extremes, or drastic measures to make changes happen. It was planned, calculated, and a slow enough process where my mind and body were working together. In my previous competition, my body changed drastically, but my mind did not. That stark contrast left me worse than when I started.

It inspired me to bring my creativity into the kitchen and look for new challenges. Looking back at my old eating habits, I realized I didn't have to give anything up. I just had to take an alternate approach to incorporate more of the foods I loved. It was completely possible to make them fit my new lifestyle using Flexible Dieting. I wasn't willing to sacrifice taste, cravings, or certain foods, and this forced me to get creative and work my macro magic. If I wanted to eat something but found that the macros didn't fit my caloric budget, I'd adjust the recipe to make it more macro-friendly.

For example, I found a recipe for a Mocha Chocolate Icebox Cake, which called for heavy cream, soft cheese, cookies, chocolate chips—all the dressings and replicated it. I swapped out heavy cream with a milk substitute, soft cheese with fat-free cream cheese, reduced the number of cookies, and added in a protein powder to thicken the batter. One holiday, I made a protein cheesecake and took it to a family gathering, and no one could tell the difference—it was that good! I've always loved experimenting with new recipes and tapping into my creative side, and I fell in love with the fun of the challenge.

The great thing about Flexible Dieting is that it really is flexible. You can customize and flex it to fit your lifestyle.

Growing up, I didn't care much for breakfast, except for Saturday mornings. On Friday evenings, my mother would grocery shop after work. Once home, we'd tear through the bags like it was Christmas morning just to see what cereal she'd surprised us with. This would determine our Saturday morning plans and set off sibling rivalry.

After setting our alarm clocks, my brothers and I would race downstairs to claim dibs on the *good* cereal; first come, first served. The winner selected their choice and claimed the prize inside the box. Still, to this day, Cocoa Pebbles or Lucky Charms are a staple in my house. Nowadays, I love breakfast. It's the meal I most look forward to. And not because it's the first, but because it's a fresh start to use my creative talents and a fun way to express myself through art and science.

I would never consider myself a good cook, but making something on-the-fly gave me a feeling of accomplishment. I was good at it, and it fueled my confidence while I was in my creative zone. When you're good at something you love to do, you do it with passion and confidence while taking pride in yourself. I never knew this sense of accomplishment, paired with happiness, existed.

I felt others had the right to that feeling, as did the people I envied and compared myself to, always wondering why they had what I didn't. I was looking everywhere for this answer but never sought the wisdom within. I needed to see it to believe it.

Having a healthy attitude about food and nutrition allowed me to overcome my food fears and anxieties. It gave me food freedom. I now saw food as fuel to nourish my body, mind, and soul. I felt fulfilled, healthy, and balanced. To this day, I still practice moderation and live a healthy, balanced diet. There are days when I enjoy more, but that's life. I just move on to the next day—no need to live in the past, locked in old fears or obsessions. I'd rather keep moving forward. I call this progress.

I started to see the visual transformation as my body began to change. I had so much momentum that I took full advantage and rode the high. There was no stopping me! It was the best I'd ever been.

During this competition prep, I made sure to include people, events, and daily life with balance and moderation. It wasn't about how much I could exclude or sacrifice, but rather how much could I include or gain while I worked toward my goals.

Chuck and I never missed our date night. I looked forward to my weekly refeed day, a temporary increase in calories designed to boost my leptin levels and help me feel fuller longer. We'd plan an evening to include fun foods like pizza and ice cream. Even though my daily macros got cut leading up to the show, we managed to continue our date nights.

I learned and practiced variations of Flexible Dieting. For example, on date nights, I'd eat protein and vegetables throughout the day, saving the bulk of my carbs and fat calories for dinner. Another option is by extending the periods between meals—intermittent fasting. For example, skipping breakfast and eating my first meal around 1:00 p.m. and another meal around 9:00 p.m. I prefer spacing meals further apart throughout the day to enjoy larger portions and to stay fuller longer. Although there are many different ways to *flex* or *fast*, it's best to find what works for you, your lifestyle, and your health and fitness goals.

Flexible Dieting and Intuitive Eating

Flexible Dieting is the key to food freedom. It follows the belief that there are no foods off-limits, creating a sustainable and flexible approach to dieting, one of balance, and moderation. Flexible Dieting helps create new habits, food beliefs, and focus on nutrition. It encourages one to get over fears of labels and food myths such as good/bad, healthy/junk, clean/dirty. To reach your nutrition goals, it helps to develop habits you can measure by collecting data and by weighing, tracking, and logging your food intake. This way, you're able to manage what and how much you consume.

The more you practice, the more you'll learn, understand, and reap the benefits of having flexibility in your diet. You'll reach a place of less reliance on weighing, tracking, and logging food. You're able to go about social events and daily living by identifying portion control and portion size. Wise food choices are based on nutritional value. It's your choice whether or not you want to log or track macro data. Through

the practice and process, you'll uncover another benefit—
Intuitive Eating.

Intuitive Eating is being fully in tune with your mind and
body. You listen, feed, nourish, and fuel the body, when and
with what it needs. You eat when hungry and stop when fully
satisfied. Foods are chosen for their ability to satisfy first and
foremost, not because of any dietary guidelines. That's because
by this time you know which foods to avoid—trigger foods.
If you feel like eating a heaping bowl of Lucky Charms, you
don't label it as bad or bingeing. You do *you*—no regrets, no
self-sabotage, no reverting back to eating disorders or body
dysmorphia.

The practice of macro tracking, from a nutritional
standpoint, taught me to choose my food wisely and to choose
whole foods over-processed. Macro tracking changed how
I ate and looked at food altogether. Throughout the entire
process, from Flexible Dieting to Intuitive Eating, I tuned
into my body and how it responded to various foods.

Some foods agree with me more than others. I no longer
have a gallbladder; I've learned what trigger foods to avoid.

Being entirely in sync with mind and body will allow you
to recognize when, where, how, and why you eat. You will
know when to eat, and you'll hear your mind signal you to
stop eating. That's why it's called Intuitive Eating. I no longer
have food anxiety, and my previous eating disorders—binging,
starving, restricting, excessive workouts, and laxatives—are all
in the past. Intuitive Eating has allowed me to create a healthy
relationship with food, mind, and body. I enjoy what I eat
and eat what I enjoy with balance and moderation, creating
a lifestyle that best serves me.

Emotional eating was something of the past. I ate to fill a void. Now I can ask myself questions like: *Am I hungry or bored? Is it that time of the month again? Why am I mindlessly eating? What am I trying to fill or accomplish?* When I recognize the emotional triggers behind these questions, I can then control my responses and food choices.

* * *

In a competition, you don't get a gold star, credit, or a trophy for how hard you suffered or how you stuck perfectly to your meal plan or hit your macros. Even if you don't hit these targets, what matters is knowing who you are and why you are entering the show.

The true win is in having a stable mindset and bouncing back from setbacks. When you're grounded in who you are, you become *Unstoppable*. Find a balance that works for you and do whatever it is with passion and purpose.

I took this advice from my former self and incorporated it into my last competition. It was all about me. I didn't suffer, sacrifice, or give anything up. In fact, I gained so much it overshadowed the competition and became a sport I was passionate about again. I love to live life, lift weights, and eat. I showed up on stage, reflecting my passions—all glammed up.

Seeking approval from others brought me into the competitive sport of bodybuilding. In 2012, I allowed strangers to judge me and used my body as a means to determine my worth. It didn't go as planned, and I ended up further down in a pit of self-doubt and self-loathing for years. Today, I have a new love for fitness and health as a lifestyle, not a destination. Through the process of self-care and self-love, I learned how to truly love and respect myself—so much so that I'm now able to be an example to others. I never imagined people would see me as inspiration. As a result, my life has become one I am proud of: a life of joy and happiness. Far from perfection—whatever that word even means now—my life is clear and simplified.

Trying to balance this new me, mentally, physically, emotionally, and spiritually was a daily challenge. I worked on these areas simultaneously, and while they were important individually, they were so much more powerful in full alignment. If I'd give in to my old ways of thinking, the consequence would have been the miserable, self-hating life I'd worked so hard to escape. I had to stick to a new set of beliefs, values, routines, habits, behaviors, and more. It wasn't easy and still isn't even today. I am a continual work in progress. Through self-awareness, I've learned to manage my responses differently.

Inherently, our foundations are passed down from generation to generation, but it's up to us to change what doesn't work. It's up to us to create a legacy, a new story. Even though you want to change, moments of relapse are very common. The difference between then and now is awareness and how you choose to respond or react. It's about resilience, how long it takes for you to recognize a mistake, and how quickly you can correct the behavior and get back on track. Still, unresolved emotional blocks required attention. For me, that place was my home.

Along the Way: Declutter and Prioritize

I started decluttering, getting rid of what was draining my energy and weighing me down. First to go were my five-hour drives to visit *home* in Buffalo. It wasn't filling me. Over the years, I'd made it easy for others to see me by inserting myself into their lives. As the long drives started to take a toll on me, I reasoned it was easier for me to go to them instead of having them come to me. It took me many years to thoroughly understand my wants. I realized I needed *them* more than they needed *me*. That's why they didn't visit me. Once I became aware of this, I was able to replace my need by building a life of my own in Columbus. If anyone wanted to see me, they knew where I lived.

Change is often painful at first, and I had moments where I longed to continue my visits to Buffalo, but for me to grow and learn, I needed to endure the short-term pain of nostalgia and disappointment and replenish that emotional deficit with a new life here in Columbus.

With that, I opened my heart and mind to connect with like-minded individuals, starting with my gym and with Meetup.com. I was reluctant to plant roots in my city and community, based on a series of lies, limiting beliefs, and excuses, over the many years I'd lived there. It was very much about me and what was in it for me. I had not poured anything into my city, yet I expected that the people would pour into me. For me to meet and connect with new people, I needed to be physically present and plant roots. I was yearning for a sense of belonging in Columbus, a place for me to call my home. But I wasn't ready and willing to be open or to feel a connection.

What you are looking for is also looking for you. I found individuals whom I valued and developed relationships with them. I connected in ways I never could before. I finally felt like I belonged. A yoga class offered at my gym drew me in. Ironically, it was called Yin, the opposite of my yang strength-training. Even more ironic, they later renamed it

Surrender. Surrender had been a buzz word I'd ignored. At first, as I began slowing down, letting go, giving up, I learned to surrender.

Initially, I found it challenging to quiet my mind while stretching my beaten body. Through the practice, I found peace in the silence, and comfort in the discomfort. I learned to enjoy and observe the thoughts and voices in my head while resisting the urge to dwell on them. Instead, I acknowledged them and let them pass by. If you don't listen to those voices, they have no one to talk to, and the thoughts move on as quickly as they appeared. I let the thoughts go.

While on my mat, holding these uncomfortable and excruciating poses, the instructor would share stories and parables, teaching us a lesson and shifting our attention from the pain and discomfort. Whatever you focus on will grow, so those stories were the perfect diversion.

Through my weekly yoga practice, I began to get comfortable with my thoughts. My alone time on the mat reaped serious conversations and real talk with self. Week after week, these self-dialogues grew deeper and more meaningful, and I began to enjoy my own company. I developed a relationship with myself on a more profound level, one I'd never known before. I got to know *me*.

I'd leave my mat and class feeling refreshed and relaxed, as if I'd just had a mental massage. Something changed on that yoga mat. *I had changed.* It was during those moments of silence and shifting my thoughts inward that I could answer such fundamental questions as: *Who am I? What's holding me back? Why is it holding me back?*

Now, I challenge you to sit and ask yourself these same questions. Can you answer these questions with honesty and conviction? No matter what your personal, professional, fitness, or health desires are, if you don't ask and answer these fundamental questions for yourself, you will not gain the insight necessary to create a life uniquely your own.

Can you ask these questions while looking at yourself in the mirror, imperfections and all? Instead of focusing on the flaws and awakening the inner voice for a critical conversation, simply acknowledge them without judgment and extend yourself some grace. We are all imperfect. Remember that what you consider flaws are someone else's ideal of beauty. It's all about perception. When we have self-love and a deep sense of who we are, we're able to view ourselves and the world at large from a place of love and compassion. The alternative is anger, hate, and destruction—the opposite of living.

Let's change the way we see ourselves, and the way we see ourselves will change. We will experience a newfound feeling of self-love. It's what's in our hearts that's most important. We are so much more than our reflections in the mirror. This body we see, it's more than vanity. It's a vehicle, a tool of great purpose. It's a medium by which we attain our higher calling and find our purpose for living (i.e., giving and serving selflessly through love and compassion).

If you are continually living your life the way you think others want you to, what's its purpose and whom does it serve? I've often found that we're asking for permission and seeking validation and acceptance from others. We've allowed our societal norms, rules, expectations, parents, friends, family, surroundings, and our past to define us. We look to others, to see if it's okay to embrace and love ourselves as we are.

Loving yourself and having confidence doesn't make you prideful, arrogant, egotistical, conceited, or whatever judgy word you want to attach to it. To use those words and labels against yourself in such a negative way disempowers you and is a complete disservice to yourself and others. Those who do take offense and feel the need to label others—well, that's on them. Perhaps their judgments and attempt at controlling you stem from insecurity or envy, and they wish they had what you have. Regardless, it's up to you to take your power back, be an inspiration, and empower others to do the same. Keep in mind, everyone hurts, and everyone struggles. Every person responds differently. Some may become defensive, perceiving an attack on their own ego and may react in retaliation by name-calling or belittling your achievements. Our words have power.

I hadn't learned how to love and accept myself or to embrace myself with confidence in a way I understood. When I saw others filled with love and confidence, I wanted it and resented them for having it and being what I wanted to be. Feeling hurt and jealous, I belittled them, which also limited and diminished myself.

While I still fall victim to negative self-talk, I choose not to stick around to chat with it. I've learned to hear it and not listen. I know what the truth is versus the lies it's told me in the past.

Having self-awareness allowed me to realize that everything is a choice. There are days I'll stare at myself in the mirror, looking for new ways to love myself, and my eyes will immediately go to my areas of insecurity. I scrutinize my thick lower body and newly sprouted gray hairs. At this moment, I have a choice. Do I entertain these negative thoughts, feed into them, believe them, and allow them to consume my thoughts and energy? Do I allow this knowing I cannot change the structure of my body or defy aging? Allowing destructive thoughts will lead to more self-sabotage and ruin my day. It will also affect those around me because of the negative attitude it creates. I will be down, sad, and hurt, and it will cause a ripple effect.

Instead of spiraling down a negative path, I merely take notice, acknowledge the areas I cannot control, and move on with love, acceptance, and gratitude. I am alive. I am more than this body. I have a purpose of empowering myself and others. My wish is for you to become your best self. I encourage you to let go of your limiting beliefs, and to redefine who you are. I urge myself to focus on what I do have, not on what I don't. I urge you to do the same. You have more than you realize.

Today, I create a loving list instead of a loathing list. It's easier said than done, and I didn't arrive here overnight. It took years and a lot of practice to rewire my old thought patterns and create new habits to serve myself and those around me. The power of positive thinking and gratitude have significantly impacted my view of life and the world around me.

* * *

I attended an event and was introducing myself to people I hadn't seen since I was a child. Directly in front of me, a guest commented to my younger brother, "I didn't know you had a sister." *Yep, I'm right here. I can see and hear you.*

Immediately, I felt small and regressed to that lost child inside, and the voice in my head mocked me. *Are you kidding me? Yes, I do exist. Thanks for just now noticing!*

I swallowed my pride and smiled as I introduced myself.

The comment dug into a wound I'd been working on healing, and even though it was on the mend, I could still feel the sting. I am a work in progress and will continue to feel as I heal.

After the comment, I noticed that the change in me was obvious. I chose to respond in a positive way instead of reacting negatively out of fear and a bruised ego. With self-awareness, I turned this around by not retreating to that old familiar place. I knew who I was, and the path I was on, and finally, no one else's opinion mattered.

Points to Ponder

Identifying emotional triggers:

Do you find yourself stuck in emotional eating?

Do you tend to overeat, or do you stop when you are full?

What triggers prompt you to emotionally eat?

In what area are you focusing your energy on?

Is it on something you have or what you do not?

What is something you can add to your loving list?

What is draining the bulk of your energy?

How are you fueling yourself—physically, mentally, emotionally, and spiritually?

THIRTEEN

Go Home: Let Go and Forgive the Unforgivable

One month into 2015's competition prep, Chuck and I needed a break from each other, and I returned to Buffalo. All this inside work brought up the desire to return to the places of my childhood where I'd once felt safe and happy. This time, it was winter and the coldest month in Buffalo's history.

For a month, I stayed at an Airbnb with my cat, William. I went to the gym, the grocery store, and came back to my cozy little apartment to work. It was during this downtime of boredom and loneliness that I forced myself to sit in the ugly discomfort of my own company and ask myself the hard, honest questions I'd fought so desperately to avoid: *Who am I? Why am I here?*

During this stay, I learned that my beloved Uncle Angelo (not the abuser) had been diagnosed with cancer. In one of our many talks that month, he asked why I was in Buffalo. The question prompted a pause. I had to fess up. "I left my husband," I heard myself confess. And as much as it hurts to say those words aloud, I understood that I didn't know the fate of my marriage. My uncle shared a story about his own marriage and told me he should have tried harder to make it work.

"Go home," he told me. "Make up with your husband. You don't want to end up like me."

I'd never known this side of my uncle. I felt his pain. I began to cry for him, for myself, and for my husband.

In the month I spent apart from Chuck, I realized I had to make our home in Columbus work or else move on. I was straddling two lives, one in Buffalo and one in Columbus, and it was time to make a choice. I had rejected my husband during my years of emptiness.

When I practiced this new and radical approach to self-care, it moved me forward in my journey of self-development—personally and professionally. I discovered a hole in my spirituality like a missing piece in a jigsaw puzzle. And I knew what it was. I hadn't fully turned to God.

Once you dive into healing yourself and your spirit is ready, all areas come calling for resolution. Here, spirituality led me to surrender myself, my burdens and worries to God, and ask for forgiveness. I could not have forgiveness without faith. It was something I needed so desperately before I returned to the new competitions and life in Columbus. I needed to forgive my husband, my parents, my abuser, and everyone who I felt had wronged and harmed me. But first, I needed to learn to forgive myself.

Forgiveness does not mean you allow people a pass for their actions. Instead, it's a way of letting go. Harboring feelings of anger, bitterness, resentment, guilt, and shame confine you to a self-created prison. You can't realize your dream of who you want to be if you're stuck behind the walls of your own making.

Through my faith, and the death and resurrection of Jesus Christ, I am forgiven and made new. I live with purpose— no shame, judgment, or condemnation. My life, my worth, and my identity is found in Him, not others, and having that relationship and understanding has allowed me to become free.

I have turned my abuser over to God. He can judge and deal with him when his time comes. Who or what you choose to follow in your faith and life—whether it's Jesus, the Universe, a higher power, or divine guidance—is entirely up to you.

The separation between my husband and I gave us time and room to breathe and grow—as individuals and as a couple. Being together personally and professionally 24/7 produced a highly stressed home and work environment; it magnified everything.

I wanted control over every aspect of my life, micromanaging even the most mundane and minute details, easily aggravated me. Our dog's constant need for attention was one example. *Stop moving! Can't you just lay still?!* Oh, and the barking? Don't even get me started!

I wasted countless hours and energy trying to shift, control, and do whatever I could to make everything fit my idea of perfection. My expectations were unrealistic, but, damn it, I was determined to make it work! Maybe I needed to do more, be more, try harder in my constant, draining quest to be *enough*.

The more I lost control, the more bitter and angry I'd become, adding to the crumbling foundation we built our marriage upon. I needed a break. I couldn't do this anymore, for neither myself nor my husband. It was during my break in Buffalo that I could step back, gain some clarity, and take personal responsibility for myself and my actions. I had no one but myself to blame for the choices and decisions in my life. I was the reason my life was out of control. I was resisting the natural flow.

What you resist will still persist. No wonder life wasn't changing. I wasn't allowing it to change. I needed to let go, to surrender, and let everything unfold the way it was intended.

It was much easier for me to change than to force change in the lives of everyone and everything around me. It was a lesson learned the hard way. My striving for perfection and control was one grand illusion. Life is supposed to be real, raw, and messy. (Yes, dogs bark. A lot! It's okay.)

When I returned to my marriage, I had to face the need to control my husband. Exhausted from my efforts, realizing it was much easier to change myself versus trying to change others, I embraced a new concept—letting go. I hated the cliché. How does one let go? But it was time. I had to let go of what I wanted and what I didn't want. I made a life-changing decision. I took full responsibility for myself, my actions, ultimately, my life.

No longer would I allow others to dictate the course of my life, who I was, and what I wanted. This would be all on God and me.

I committed this time to making my home in Ohio with my husband and our two furry kids, William and Rudy a priority. They all needed and loved me. And I needed them. Another positive shift forward in my mindset brought me even closer to the right state of mind for the competition.

It wasn't until I began a relationship with the one person I was afraid of most—myself—that I could view life differently. Life wasn't happening *to* me; it was happening *for* me. I just needed to reclaim the power to make my own happiness, something I'd inadvertently given to others. I needed to empower myself.

To be consistent with this newly empowered state, I really anchored myself to God, beyond judgment and forgiveness. I searched from within and shifted the focus from me to God. It was exactly what I needed to walk into the next competition.

I asked for help and surrendered my worries, burdens, struggles, and cares to God, who lifted the weight off of me. I could then move toward my purpose with clarity and guidance. The anxiety and worries of what others thought of me no longer mattered; they did not and do not define me.

Life is temporary. I have a short time here on earth, and I want to make sure I'm living for my higher calling and purpose in life.

Points to Ponder

Why is it so easy to spot beauty in others and so challenging to find our own?

Who do you think is beautiful?

Who do you admire? Why?

We have very high expectations of our families. Where and with whom do you consider yourself at *home* today?

Are you living the life you want? Are you happy and fulfilled? If not, why not? What is holding you back?

Does a higher spirit guide you? What is it calling upon you to do?

FOURTEEN

The Comeback:
Conquering Fear with Love

To fully commit to my *comeback* into the world of competition, I chose the National Physique Committee (NPC) Mike Francois Classic. It's one of the largest shows I've attended aside from the Arnold Classic, held in Columbus, Ohio. I felt great overall and had finally hit *poverty* macros—reduced macros. As my daily calories decreased, so did my macros, starting with carbs. It didn't allow me much variety or wiggle room for creativity or treats. I had to improvise by focusing on quantity over quality with volume-based foods. For example, I'd layer my plate with zucchini noodles or spaghetti squash instead of pasta or rice and top with lean meat and cheese. Eating a larger plate took me longer to finish and allowed me to go the whole day feeling full and satisfied. I had a goal, and with each bite, I could almost taste the finish line.

This short span in poverty macros was nothing new, and it'd be over soon enough. I also had Sohee to lean on. I wasn't struggling alone anymore. You don't have to be a competitor to benefit from support in training and nutrition.

If you recall, I tried to do my own workout in the gym and failed. I wanted to lift weights post-surgery, but I didn't have a guide to help me stay consistent, and I didn't believe in myself. I was also eating like crap and drinking almost every night.

As we entered Peak Week, the week leading up to the competition day, Sohee gave me a detailed daily agenda. Preparation allowed me to be stress-free. My primary focuses were on completing my workouts, hitting macros and water, perfecting my posing, managing sleep and stress levels, and making the final arrangements for my suit, tan, hair, and makeup. This time, I was actually looking forward to the weekend! I continued to stay mentally strong and positive in the days leading up to the show.

On the day of the competition, I looked at the other women up and down. They all came from different places, and I knew nothing about them or their stories. I knew they were studying me, too, in their moments of doubt and judgment. These brief moments of self-doubt could be a mental *make-it-or-break-it*. I stayed focused on my mission of taking the stage for the second time, reminding myself of who I was and why I was there. I was cautious about not letting negativity in or allowing comparison to get the best of me. I belonged here with these other women. I kept feeding my mind positive self-talk and affirmations. *Stay focused, you've got this. You can do anything! I have everything I need within me. I am strong. I am confident. I am beautiful. I am worthy. I am a child of God.*

While sitting backstage, I overheard one girl talking.

"I can't wait to eat pizza after the show," she said proudly. She saw I was looking at her.

"What's your go-to food after the show?" she asked.

I had a flashback moment, like seeing a ghost from my past, and I felt a twinge of pain. This poor girl could be me, as I recalled my Reese's binge after the last competition in 2012. I paused for a moment as I took in the question. I tried to remember if I'd deprived myself of anything during this contest prep versus 2012 when everything outside my meal plan was off-limits and caused me to spiral post-competition.

"Hmmm," I replied, "I don't have any. I ate everything I wanted."

"Are you serious?" she said.

I told her about Flexible Dieting, and she looked at me with curiosity. I explained that with Flexible Dieting, there were no food restrictions. You lacked nothing. If it didn't fit your macros, it didn't fit. It was as simple as that. "I like to think of it as setting a calorie budget," I said, "If you can't afford something, you don't eat it."

I don't remember what she looked like or where she placed, but we all deserved to be in the competition. This year, I would not be her.

I was looking at it as a competition with myself. I get to do everything I love—eat, lift, and live my life while standing on stage with all these amazing women. It didn't matter whether the ladies were on teams or had a lot of support present for them; we supported each other.

My main support came from the trust and belief in myself and the online support of Sohee. This time around, it didn't have to be hard; I didn't need the whole blood, sweat, and tears routine. I no longer needed to sacrifice my life to show how hard I'd suffered or to prove my worth. This time, I hadn't given up anything or limited myself to a minimal food meal plan—neither were fun.

Meal plans still give me anxiety. They remind me of 2012, and I don't find them realistic. Long-term dieting is also over for me. What happens when life or meals don't go as planned? How do you deal with those situations? Do you just throw your hands up in defeat? Then, do you declare, *Screw it! I already messed up my meal plan. Might as well blow off the day—and the diet for that matter!*

This time when the competition ends, there's no need to hoard the treats I missed and binge for days. The treats and food will still be there, but now it's about having a structure and working toward goals over time. After the loss in 2012, I numbed my emotions and lack of gratification by gorging myself post-competition with holiday Reese's, pizza, and wine.

In 2012, one woman said to me, "You will never be able to go back to the old way of eating." I took that as a challenge, trying to prove her wrong. *Yeah? Watch me.* I ate and ate and ate and never got repulsed. I was used to this restrict/binge cycle, and it exacerbated my previous eating disorders.

This time, in 2015, I knew there would be an exit strategy, via reverse-dieting, to prevent the same thing from happening. There would be no excessive weight gain and no more eating disorders. I had embraced eating, lifting, and living with balance and moderation.

In any competition, there's only one winner, and I just wasn't willing to lose my life again. I was determined to never go back to that scared, broken girl I once was. I had gained too much in the process of becoming who I am.

When Class A (short) bikini division lined up for the stage, I couldn't help but eye the competition again, comparing myself to those other beautiful women. But never, ever did I feel I didn't belong. I worked very hard and much smarter this time around. I deserved to be here with those women. Knowing this was only my second competition, I was still nervous but remained remarkably calm. I practiced my breathing and prayed to God for strength, courage, confidence, and grace.

I walked on stage with the other thirty-three ladies and held my own, exhibiting poise, sass, and confidence. I was mentally sound and felt comfortable in my skin. I owned myself. I looked at the judges, smiled, and reminded myself, "It's not about what they think, I've already won."

Once pre-judging was over, I felt a huge rush of relief pass through me. *I'd done it!* I faced my fears and did what I doubted I'd ever do again! And I strutted my body with confidence on stage in an itty-bitty, teeny-weeny, blinged bikini in front of hundreds of complete strangers and allowed them to judge, mock, criticize, and say whatever they wanted. I knew who I was, and I no longer allowed the memory of a loss or the past to define me.

I overcame everything I'd feared, including the odds that stood in my way. My setback was worth the comeback, and I'd done this for me! A rush came over me—wow, this is awesome! If I can do this, I really can do anything! I cheered myself on!

I skipped off stage for our break, feeling accomplished and proud of myself for how far I'd come in less than a year. For once, I looked forward to the future; I wanted it now! My husband and friends were there to support me and give me compliments, which I graciously accepted. I deserved them.

That night, returning to the show finals, I still felt amazing. I stood proudly on stage among fifty-eight other bikini competitors, rocking my body, and owning who I had become.

Although I didn't place, I celebrated inside. I knew my worth, and it was enough. Everything I believed I couldn't do, I just did them and became unstoppable in the process! I came back stronger than ever. I didn't do this competition for a win or a trophy; I did it for me. *Was my butt as tight as the girl who won? Nope,* but that was okay. I won my life back, plus more. To me, that's priceless!

I reported back to Sohee and provided her with the judges' feedback from the NPC show. She helped me develop a new plan for my next show, the following weekend, The INBF-WNBF Tri-State Natural Pro/Amateur Championship. The International Natural Bodybuilding and Fitness Federation (INBF), an amateur affiliate of the World Natural Bodybuilding Federation (WNBF). We focused on bringing me in tighter, and leaner with improved posing.

Our goal was for me to appear more confident overall, a better package. I'd used the NPC competition to overcome my fears, so this promised to be fun and easy. I just needed to walk on stage, owning everything about myself, and if I placed, that'd be a bonus.

With our new plan, Sohee and I headed into the Tri-State show tweaking some numbers. I came in tighter, leaner, and felt my best overall. I was excited and looking forward to this smaller and less intensive competition.

I remained calm and confident during practice. I'd just competed in a giant show. My warm-up the week prior had gone well, and I looked forward to everything falling into place.

Once again, I took the stage and let it all shine. My confidence received a major boost in one week—I felt different—more at ease, owning every minute, and I presented my best package ever! Again, this was about getting my life back and becoming the person I was meant to be. Since this was a much smaller show, it was hard to tell where my fellow competitors would place. I felt indifferent, yet comfortable, with the judge's decisions, and that's how I left the stage at the break.

Over the break period, people were voicing their thoughts and opinions about the competition, and I heard someone mention they had me in the top five. I immediately dismissed it and didn't want any seeds of false hope planted. But then others chimed in agreeing. I couldn't help but wonder, *Did I? Could I have actually placed?* I got excited. *How awesome would that be?* Inside, I believed it. I mean, anything was possible.

Returning that night for the show, I kept my feelings to myself. I didn't want to be disappointed or let down. I'd left all that behind in 2012. When my number wasn't announced, the realization set in—I didn't place, and my heart sank. I cried a few silent tears, not for the loss but the closure.

Any hope of actual contest-placing would have to wait for another time. Finally, the end had come to a long and arduous journey back to the stage. I wiped my tears and stood proudly at all I'd accomplished that season. I was proud and held my head high. This was the greatest achievement of them all—self-love.

An excerpt from the Judges Feedback email read: "Very pretty and sassy (good posing), good shape, nice bikini walk, improve leg leanness/conditioning, increase shoulder development, tighten up glutes."

They didn't tell me anything I didn't already know, so it wasn't a harsh surprise. I didn't take it personally or get defensive. I read the email and agreed one hundred percent with their feedback. Best of all, I wasn't a wreck after the competition.

It's exactly how I'd seen myself, my shape and frame, but now with muscular development. That's the advantage of bodybuilding; you get to shape and build your body to meet your personal goals. Now, if they'd provided feedback on my mindset, I'm pretty sure we'd both agree it was pretty solid! It's what carried me through this entire journey.

I had overcome so much. I stood proudly on that stage, knowing, trusting, and believing in myself.

The shows proved my newfound love and a healthy relationship with food and fitness. I didn't have any rebound weight gain from either show and sat comfortably five to eight pounds heavier without fear. I have learned to love, embrace, and accept myself, and found I prefer my off-season body more. It's healthier, stronger, and I'm fully comfortable in my own skin.

Some of the biggest takeaways from the 2015 competitions were facing and overcoming fears and limitations. I did so by learning, evolving, and returning home with a refined awareness of myself.

No longer am I held back by self-limiting beliefs. No longer am I the little girl whose life had been stolen, who played small, and was desperate for love and attention. That little girl felt invisible, worthless, and needed others to define and validate her. No longer do I feel lost, alone, confused, angry, rejected, and broken. The journey, sure as hell wasn't easy by any means, as I learned to live by beliefs contrary to all the ones I previously held. I taught myself to become the very person I never believed I could be.

In terms of competing, I wasn't in it for the long term or the pro card. I didn't know it at the time, but the competition was a foundation for something bigger, and I used the stage to accomplish it.

Fitness saved my life. It was a catalyst for discovering who I was. Using fitness as an outlet, I healed my body, mind, and soul. It became my therapy.

Through strength training and bodybuilding, I created a body I love and respect. I am comfortable with who I am—most of the time. We are never one hundred percent satisfied every minute of our lives. What use is the journey without a few reminders of where you came from?

Would I consider my mind and body to be perfect according to the ideal I'd been chasing my entire life? Did I finally reach that goal? Absolutely not! But I now view my body from a place of gratitude and love. It's taken a lifetime to get to this point, to move forward from my old patterns of self-hate and self-abuse to a place of self-love and self-worth. Those whom I needed most in my life taught me to love myself. When I'd almost given up, people like my brother, John, my trainer, Sohee, and other women who'd made it through gave me confidence and courage when I lacked it. They gave me strength where I was weak. As I evolved and grew, I knew that I had to be more of a student than a teacher.

Points to Ponder

What's something huge you've accomplished, knowing you wouldn't win, but that there was something greater to gain?

What's a moment you can recall where you've pushed beyond your comfort zone?

How have you overcome your fears and embraced growth?

What are a few takeaways you can reflect on from the experience of challenging yourself?

Whatever the mind can conceive and believe, it can achieve.
—Napoleon Hill

FIFTEEN

The Gift:
Finding the Silver Lining

A week post-competition, my husband and I set off again for our anniversary vacation to Maui. This time, we were in a better place with our marriage, and there were no physical injuries to interrupt our time together. Mentally, I was still on a high coming through my competition experience.

The last few months had been a whirlwind and left me feeling a sense of overwhelming gratitude. I felt so blessed. Looking back at the accomplishments of 2015, I gave glory to God for making all of this possible. I'd had a second chance, a do-over from 2012. I had walked through a lifetime of healing and self-discovery in three years.

My calories were still low, but I knew what enjoying every bit of my vacation entailed: food freedom. I wanted to indulge without feelings of guilt or shame, but I also knew I needed a plan, a framework to live by to avoid the downward spiral following my 2012 competition. I voiced my worries and concerns to Sohee, and she prepared me for my exit from the competitions. She introduced me to reverse dieting, and slowly and methodically added calories back into my plan up to my body's maintenance level. It would allow me to achieve my personal goals.

Reverse dieting was an entirely new concept for me. In fact, it was a relatively new term in the fitness industry and something I should have been introduced to and made aware of in 2012 before I sabotaged myself.

Although I'd created a solid plan and had a great relationship with my coach, I knew I had to let go and trust in the process. Still, I couldn't help but fear the unknown. I had moments of weakness, playing the *what if* game, filling my mind with worries and doubt. *What if I gained all the weight back? What if I consumed too much in the short period, post-competition? What if I do more damage to my body?*

Throughout the sixteen weeks of reverse dieting, I slowly added in more calories, created new recipes, and enjoyed a summer filled with family, food, friends, and fun. Once I completed my reverse diet, I took a break from counting macros as I learned to trust and listen to my body and its nutritional needs.

As I progressed with learning and mastering Flexible Dieting, I gradually transitioned to Intuitive Eating. I learned to flex and stretch my food intake to fit my goals and lifestyle while accommodating and enjoying special events with balance and moderation. Being in sync with my body allowed me to eat when I was hungry and stop when I was full and satiated. I listened to what my body needed, and guilt no longer figured into the equation. This allowed me to create a lifestyle with food freedom.

After both competitions, my strength training and protein intake remained my primary goal. Even though I practiced Intuitive Eating (i.e. not tracking or using a food journal), I was fully aware (being mindful of what I was eating). This was, in part, because I ate the same way I did for contest prep, including foods I loved, just more of them.

Thankfully, my mindset was sound enough to offset the waves of fear and doubt. I had the power to control my choices and practice everything I'd learned since working with Sohee. I wanted to enjoy my vacation without feeling like I was on a diet. So, I fully embraced and trusted that she knew what was best for me. I had worked so hard to get to this mental and physical place where I could eat, lift, and live my life in balanced harmony. And I did just that for the first thirty-six hours we were in Maui. Then the call came, Uncle Angelo, my mother's brother, had passed away.

The last time I saw Uncle Angelo was three months ago. He'd just learned of his cancer. I hadn't expected him to pass away so soon.

The time I spent in Buffalo had a greater purpose, a gift I could never replace. My uncle and I spent quality one-on-one time together. Knowing I could be there with him and for him gave my trip home a deeper sense of meaning and purpose. In retrospect, it was about more than taking a break from my husband. It was providence, an opportunity to be there for my Uncle Angelo and he for me. We were two broken people knowing our lives were about to drastically change.

I recalled that the hours spent with my uncle, our off-the-wall conversations, laughter, and good times brought a smile to his face in that dark time. But the gift he gave me, the example of strength and humor, was even more profound. It was a memory and an experience I will never forget.

When he told me, "Go home, make up with your husband, you don't want to end up like me," I sat there, feeling helpless. I remember thinking, *If only I could do more for him and this situation . . . but what can I do?*

This moment had forced me to face it with truth and clarity. Empathy and compassion allowed me to see things from a different perspective. No longer was it about me. I had to get outside myself and ask, *What can I do for him?*

Uncle Angelo was the link to home that taught me not to take my husband and life in Ohio for granted. Leaving my own demons behind to be of service to my beloved uncle was exactly what I needed to reset my priorities.

After the call, I slipped out onto the balcony before the sun rose and listened to the waves crash upon the shore. I felt peace wash over me and thanked God for the special gift of our time and conversations together. Without my Uncle Angelo's sage advice, I might not be here, on another anniversary vacation with my husband. Chuck woke a short time later, and I had to break the bad news. He held and comforted me, asking what I needed, and we started planning our flight back to Buffalo.

With the continued support of Chuck and my post-competition nutrition plan from Sohee, they provided me with the proper tools during this stressful time. I stayed the course in Maui and in Buffalo. I had zero rebounds.

Points to Ponder

What are some ways you're able to find the silver lining in a difficult situation?

What changes can you make to create a lifestyle of food freedom?

How can you cultivate a lifestyle of more peace, joy, love, and happiness?

How can you spend more time being present and enjoy the moments with loved ones?

SIXTEEN

F'it! The Power of Our Words

While I've been willing to share what worked for me and what didn't, there is no one-size-fits-all antidote. I found my way by surrendering, asking for help, and trusting others. I wanted to create a lifestyle that I could take pride in. I wanted to create a loving and nurturing relationship with myself, my husband, and others, and a healthier and positive relationship with fitness and nutrition.

I am a work in progress not only physically but mentally, emotionally, and spiritually as well. Having a connection to my higher calling has allowed me to focus on my purpose of serving others. I have developed a mindset that positively feeds my thoughts and has enabled me to become my best self. I now care for my physical body—the vehicle that transports me to fulfill my purpose and to inspire, encourage, and empower others to do the same.

Spiritual Fitness

My spiritual journey took a lot of growth and nurturing. It wasn't just about prayer. It was prayer married to action, even if I wasn't sure of myself. I was loved. All I needed was to love myself. That was the first non-negotiable I committed to—I had to love, honor, and respect myself in the highest regard before I could love, honor, and respect others. Although it's taken me a lifetime to learn this lesson, my mother was right. "You have to be your own best friend first before you can be someone else's."

Regarding God, it's not easy to love, trust, and believe in a being you've neither physically seen or have a million questions about. *Who is God? Is there even a God? Is this the "right" God?* In this world, I know from personal experience and having faith that I can't do life alone. Faith does not come from seeing but hearing and believing there is a higher power much greater than myself.

I'll never forget a conversation I had with one of my friends, who was also a mentor when I was feeling stuck. At the time, I was struggling with a situation, and I asked her for help. Honestly, what I wanted was for her just to tell me what to do. Instead, she challenged and questioned why I was resistant to making a final decision.

"I don't feel confident in making this decision on my own," I said.

"Why?"

"Because they won't understand it," I replied, growing frustrated and wondering if this had been a bad idea.

"Why?"

"Because it sounds stupid." I was digging for reasons now.

"Why?"

I could feel the heat rise within me as my irritation with her grew. "Because I don't know how to do it."

"Why do you think you don't know how to do it?" she asked softly.

"Because I'm stupid!" I yelled. "What if I do it wrong?"

"Why would you do it wrong?"

I felt a part of me weaken. I was coming apart and started to let my guard down. Slowly, the hard exterior was melting in the presence of my mentor, who cared enough to stay in this conflict with me. Aside from my husband, no one had stuck with me this long through one of my spells of self-doubt.

"Because if I do it wrong, it'll prove I am stupid, and I am a failure. And if I am a failure, I'll never be good enough." There. I'd said it. Aloud to a witness.

"So what?" she replied, knowing that was the real, honest answer she was looking for. My mentor and I used a process I call *Mind Funneling*. It forced me to get clear about my intentions—freeing myself from doubt. I had all the answers inside of me already. But when I was afraid to make a final decision, she helped navigate a path for me.

By asking question after question, she created a mind funnel that reached down to the root of my actions and reasoning, forcing me to face the pain and fears I kept locked inside. This allowed me to funnel back up with answers that best served my intent, expectations, and goals to create a new foundation of beliefs and choices.

We all avoid admitting our deepest fears because, well, let's face it, they're scary and ugly. We turn to distractions and use diversions and misdirection to dance around the truth of our inner selves. Knowing so much more about my mind and body, I urged myself not to fall back to my old denials but to find someone to hold me to my intentions—whether it was in the gym or in life.

After this exchange with my mentor, I felt like I'd just hit a brick wall, head-on! *She was right!* So what if I failed? Failure doesn't define me. I'd failed many times. Shame was so familiar; I couldn't recognize it as a source. Instead, it became my identity. I even considered my 2012 competition a failure when it was, in actuality, a victory. It was hardly a loss. It sent me to a bottom from which I found the reserves to claw my way up and get help. Where I had been at fault was allowing the *what if* conversations to play over and over again instead of just allowing myself to be enough. You'll never know what's in store for you unless you challenge your fears.

All too often, we play small and live in the confines of self-made prisons because of potential criticism, rejection, failures, and ultimately, our fear of not being enough. Fear is crippling and paralyzing, which is why so many of us protect ourselves and live safely behind the walls we've built.

Everything you desire is waiting for you beyond those walls—growth, opportunity, connection, belonging, and love.

Mind Funneling

Even small decisions and awareness of your daily actions can be opportunities to drill down further and understand why you like what you like. You can then decide whether to accept it or change it, and that's one of the key benefits to mind funneling.

This process works with any question in human behavior. I often use this practice on myself to understand why I do what I do or to discover what's triggering my wants, needs, and desires. I believe our decisions come down to two desires: What am I trying to lose or gain? Am I running away from fear or towards love?

I tested this process and amazed myself at how many layers I had to peel back to get to the root of my actions. For example, I found myself in the snack aisle at Target mindlessly grabbing a package of *A Handful of Everything* trail mix. When I got home, I opened the bag and started picking through the items I didn't care for like raisins, coconut flakes, and almonds. I really only wanted the banana chips and apricots. As I looked at the pile of stuff included in the *everything*, I asked myself, "Why do I continue to buy this if I'm just going to sort through and pick just the fruit?" Also, the *everything* I was picking out ruined the flavor of what I wanted most—the banana chips. *So, why don't I just buy banana chips? Why am I conditioned to get this snack?* I had to drill down, mind-funnel, and ask, "What's really going on here?"

By funneling down, I could identify the cause. As a small child, I spent many weekends visiting my grandparents in the city. One highlight of the weekend was shopping at the big grocery store. It was a treat compared to the small country stores near where I lived. Papa would let us choose snacks from the bulk section, and I would get banana chips. He liked them as well. It was this deep-down memory, a loving one, that fueled the decision to pick up the bag of *A Handful of Everything* to get to the banana chips. I had convinced myself that to get what I wanted; I had to deal with the burden of everything else I didn't want. It had to be work. Subconsciously, I was trying to recreate the love and attention I once had with Papa. I conditioned myself to believe I had to fight to get love and not go directly for what I wanted—the banana chips!

You may not be asking yourself these micro-questions yet, but I assure you that if you follow the path of exploring the real reasons for your choices, you'll be amazed. You'll become curious about *you* and the discovery of your inner self.

Not knowing how to change and trying to do everything on my own hadn't worked. I needed to go against everything I believed to create something that worked for me. I took control of myself, created a new blueprint, a new set of beliefs and values along with new habits and behaviors, and the result was a new me. If I drifted in the wrong direction for a little while, that was okay. I just needed to keep moving.

Asking for help was one of the best decisions I've ever made. I outsourced the parts of my life that I no longer felt necessary to do alone. By giving myself permission to ask and receive help, I learned to develop a deeper connection within myself. I arrived at a place where I could impart all I'd learned in life and the aftermath of my first competition.

One aftermath was what I experienced by not facing up to my sexual abuse. Another was the courage it took to stay in my marriage. Today, our marriage is at its best. We have survived our hardest times together, which has strengthened us as one. We don't have a perfect marriage, but we always find a way to work through our problems and take care of each other.

You Are Not Meant to Do Life Alone

No longer do I need to feel the pressure of learning and achieving everything on my own. I hired coaches, sought mentors, talked to teachers, and opened up to my family. Asking for help is a sign of growth, not a sign of weakness. We all need help in reaching our goals and dreams. Life is not meant to be done alone. Surrender and ask for help. In my case, I needed to reclaim the power of my identity. I needed to ask myself, *Who am I? What's holding me back? Why?*

Once we identify our triggers, we then ask ourselves, *why?* When we uncover the whys to our fears and roots, we can then heal by letting go of the past, redefining who we are, and create a new story. We must face our fears and get comfortable being uncomfortable. For me, since fear often resembles anxiety, I learned to flip the script. No longer do I tell myself I am afraid, but I am excited. Recognizing the triggers has allowed me to know when I'm on the brink of something big! It's just a matter of identifying and pushing past the fears and beliefs. And in most instances, it's just a step away.

While working on myself, I found there were many women also going through similar struggles—overcoming fears, accepting their bodies, and adapting to how they view themselves.

I believe all such women can accomplish this—not by forcing fitness regimes that aren't suited to them—but by conquering their fears and embracing love. Love conquers all, and once a solid foundation of self-love is built, they can become the best versions of themselves. This chain of support is unstoppable, from one woman to another, can create unshakable confidence for all women.

We can incorporate fitness into all aspects of life, creating enjoyment, confidence, and empowerment. We can use it for much more than just meeting a goal to be skinny, sexy, or some form of external gratification.

We can all build community and can never have too much support. The more we listen to what we should do with our bodies, the more we can empower others to take the right path for themselves. Fitness was the right path for me. So many women tie their identities to fitness and nutrition and let it define them and determine their worth. You can either let it destroy you, or you can let it teach you.

If I'd had someone to show me the *hows and whys* early on, perhaps my journey wouldn't have been so arduous. There was no need to suffer as I did for as long as I did. If you're reading this book, please feel free to take my life, mishaps, and experiences, and use them as a shortcut to create something far greater for yourself. Shorten the learning curve. There is hope and a future that serves your best self in living a purpose-driven life.

Through this journey, my pain became my purpose, and my mess became my message. There is something bigger and better waiting for you beyond the limits of fear. I'm only offering what worked for me. Life consists of learning, growing, giving, and serving. In doing so, you will find yourself and what works best for you. Give back and pay it forward.

If you've been suffering for twenty-five years, ten years, or only three years, it's already too long to hold yourself back from a life of joy, love, and happiness with the body that is you. You can indeed embrace the body that you have with self-love and respect.

Strength training helped in the discovery and recovery of finding my true self. It was the perfect embodiment of my struggles, values, disappointments, and joys. And it still is the ideal fitness program uniquely suited to me … who I am as Rachel.

You can discover the fitness program that's right for you. Fitness can be part of your therapy, connecting and bringing your body, mind, and soul into alignment. While at the gym, listening to my beats, I can feel the energy and emotions move through me. I escape into a world of my own, conquering and quieting the voices, beliefs, and doubts within. It's a form of meditation. In these moments, I am who I am—strong, confident, fearless, and empowered.

This body, this vessel, like a well-oiled machine, must be cared for through proper exercise, nutrition, and rest. If you're not at your best, you cannot perform your life's purpose at its best. The purpose of telling my story is to help people become their best selves through the practice of creating a positive mindset, a healthy body, and a soul filled with self-love, self-acceptance, gratitude, and forgiveness.

Fitness isn't a one-size-fits-all solution. Don't discard whatever activity you're passionate about, whether it's running, hiking, yoga, or swimming. Weights may not be right for you, just like running wasn't for me. I'm suggesting that you approach the fitness you enjoy in a smarter, wiser way that works for you. The clearer your fitness path, the more you'll be able to sustain and enjoy it. With clarity comes freedom in food, fitness, faith, family, and friends.

Everything you need in life is already within you. You have the power, the mindset, the systems, the resources, and although you may have confronted the past, there's always more work to do. I didn't like who I was, so I became who I am today.

You have the opportunity to elevate yourself to a new level of confidence. Life is a journey, not a destination. Be patient, be still, and be in the present moment. Love and enjoy who you are; there will never ever be another person as uniquely gifted, talented, or as beautiful as you are. Own it and know your worth. You have the power to create your own story.

Today, I know I am Rachel.

Who are you?

Points to Ponder

What has changed your outlook by reading this book?

Are you thinking about your purpose in life? Do you know what it is?

Are you ready for change?

Is there a reason or an excuse that you use for not asking for help?

Be honest. No one's going to judge you.

If your dream doesn't scare you, it's too small.
—Mark Batterson

Acknowledgments

Thank you, God, for making all things new and possible. For teaching me how to love and for showing me who I am and whose I am.

Thank you to Sohee Lee for being a mentor, providing support, encouragement, accountability, and, most importantly, for believing in me.

A special thank you to my book coach, Kim O'Hara, who helped me make this book and my story possible. Thank you for believing in me, Kim, and for sitting with me through the journey of pain and healing with compassion and empathy.

Thank you to my husband, Chuck, who allowed me to share our deepest, darkest moments in this book. Although they were painful to re-live, without them, we wouldn't have our story or the marriage we have now. Thank you, Chuck, for never giving up and believing in me when I didn't believe in myself. Thank you for your unconditional love and support. I am blessed to call you my husband.

Thank you to my brothers Jason, Jeremy, and John. Your continuous love, encouragement, and support have been my rocks.

Lastly, but most importantly, my parents, Ross and Maria, thank you. There are no words to express my gratitude and appreciation for all you have done. Thank you for being the pillars of our family. Even when it was hard, you always did your best. Thank you for being examples, for the constant support and endless amounts of love, patience, forgiveness, and grace you've given. Thank you for allowing me to know you, to hear your stories, to sit with you in the deepest and darkest moments of our lives—the loss of your son and my brother. Thank you for being spiritual mentors and leaders, instilling in me the Christian faith. Growing up wasn't easy. On the outside, we were a modest household, but on the inside, we had more than enough—we had love. For this, I am forever grateful and wouldn't change a single thing. Because of you, I am Rachel. Thank you. I love you.

The End

Notes

1   *Clueless.* Directed by Amy Heckerling. Hollywood: Paramount Pictures. 1995

2   *What's Eating You* "Adrienne & Danni." Directed by Kathryn Douglas. E! Entertainment Television. October 13, 2010

3   Ruiz, Miguel. *The Four Agreements: A Practical Guide to Personal Freedom.* San Rafael, CA: Amber-Allen Pub. 1997.

4   Drake. "Best You Ever Had." *So Far Gone.* Young Money/ Cash Money Records, Released February 13, 2009.

5   Eminem. "Beautiful." *Relapse.* Aftermath Entertainment, 2009, Released August 11, 2009.

6   Lee, Sohee. "Sohee Fit." 2019, https://www.soheefit.com

7   *The Stepford Wives.* Directed by Frank Oz. Hollywood: Paramount Pictures and Dreamworks Pictures. 2004.

About the Author

Rachel is a Fitness and Lifestyle Enthusiast, Entrepreneur, Author, Speaker, and Host of *The Confident Woman Podcast*. She helps empower women to get fit from within by challenging and inspiring women to let go of their limiting beliefs, redefine who they are, and create their own story. As a part of her mission, Rachel has taken years of fears, failures, setbacks, and extreme loss and created simple, yet powerful, lessons that help women transform their lives and become their best and most confident selves. Rachel resides in Columbus, Ohio with her husband.

For more, visit www.iamrachelbrooks.com

Made in the USA
Middletown, DE
14 July 2021